Conversations from Room 1170

Dave Johnson

Copyright © 2018 Dave Johnson

All rights reserved.

ISBN-13: 978-1719324441

ISBN-10:1719324441

With Much Gratitude

To Dr. Van De Bruyn, for holding our hands in the dark those first years. For taking a chance.

To the Barger family, and especially to Mindi. Your great tragedy has become a touchstone for so many people. Thanks for being in the right place at the right time.

To Lisa Salberg and the HCMA. The Jersey Girl who fights HCM with bare hands and sharp tongue. You did it for Lori and it saved us. You are a light in dark places.

To our dear friends who were there at the very beginning and chose to clean theaters, drive cars, push mops, help us move, and stand behind us through that awful first year - Spencer, Tiffany, Leslie, Jason, Smitty, and our beloved Robin.

To my TTLG family near and far. You have been a shelter, a sounding board, and a refuge from storms. I love you Taffers dearly, and the fact that we all found each other in the internet ocean still boggles my mind. I wish I could list you all here individually, but I must at least mention Dia, Suzy (BA), Mara (MsLedd), Luis (Quack Quack!), Chris (RBJ), Val (V. Equinox), and my brother in arms, Alex (GBM). You know things that aren't written here because you were there from the beginning, and I know you'll be there at the end. We're awesome like that. Everything else is…well, you know.

To our Pennsylvania friends, the Arnolds, McCurdy's, Geckers, Ditzlers, Mudges, Foleys, and Frankums, who carried us when we couldn't walk or even crawl. There aren't enough pages to describe your generosity and kindness.

To our families for more than can be said here.

To Dr. Barry and Marty Maron, Dr. Harry Lever, Dr. William Allen, Dr. Mark Link, Dr. Eric Popjes, Dr. John Beohmer, Dr. David Sliber, Dr. Barry Clemson, Dr. Christoph Brehm, Dr. Dirk Pabst, Dr. Behzad Soleimani, Dr. Omaima Ali, Dr. Michael Hayes, PA-C Amy Warner, Dr. Kane High, Dr. Sarah Hussein, Dr. Octavio Falcucci, and Dr. Dwight Davis, the smartest man I've ever met. Thank you for saving my life.

To my HMC nursing team: First and foremost – to Natalie & Joanne for patience through long days and uncertainty; you have been our superheroes. To Sarah B.(I miss you!), Angie, Kelly, Krista (for carrying me), Joanna (are you trying to exsanguinate me!?), Jen, Cindy, Lori (I'm totally suing you), Mark, Big Mark, Jordan, Adam, Alex (1 & 2), Sam (1 & 2), Nona, Aileen, Ron, Mem, Jan, Beth, Andre, Kathy, Tyler, Kathleen, Beth, Allison (don't play that with your kids!), Dan (aka Ben), all the Johns, Rick, Bill, Denise (what are you reading?), Elizabeth, Liz (oh, so we're just doing this?), Erica, Brenna, Mark, Sonja, Brenna, Karen, Jena, Amy, (can you wash my hair?) Lauren, Shawn, Tommy, Brenda, Nate (this guy's trying to kill me…), Kelly, Katie (everything is still your fault), Dean in PT (for not putting up with my crap) and Jenn the PICC wizard. And to Cassie, who was there on the worst of all days. It really does take a village. I'm glad I was part of yours.

To the cath lab crew - Bill, Elizabeth, Denise (what are you reading?) Tyler, Zoe, Angel, and Rick. You all still owe me a lobster dinner.

To Ty, Jerry, and especially to Dug of King's X. Your songs are the soundtrack of my life, especially the last eight years of it. Turns out you were right; We are Still Finding Who We Are.

To Terry Pratchett, my cosmic guru. You showed me Death, sickness, God, life, and orangutans in a different light, and it kept me alive. Pardon my Klatchian, but damn do I miss you.

To that stranger on the plane in Boston, wherever you are. We never took you up on the offer to stay at your house, but you gave us hope in humanity when all else seemed dark.

To all my coordinators - Tina, Maria, Bob, Rebecca, Laura, Taylor, Alex, and Heather. And above all to Fran, who told me so. (But WHY?)

To Blake, Jamie, Jo, Dot, and James. I hope this has done you and your families what justice it can.

To Victoria, Rosie, Sam, and Holly, four of the strongest women I've ever known.

Dedications

To the 22 people who die every day waiting for a life-saving organ that never came. You are not forgotten. We who survived are still fighting for your cause. May your voices always be heard.

To Perry. It has been told, as agreed upon, the best that I can tell it. Thank you for being a big brother, our superhero, our Yoda, a reality check, and a friend. To me you'll always be Indestructible.

To Christie, Rich, and Brennan, who stood alongside me, withstood my frustration, my anger, my grief, and literally carried my life in their hands. We have done the impossible, and that makes us mighty. I love you.

And to my donor and his family. I don't know who you are, but you are with me always. Words don't solve suffering, and they cannot repay the gift I've been given. All I can do is tell anyone who will listen about your sacrifice. This is my feeble attempt to do so. Peace to you.

Forward

by

Dr. Marty Maron, M.D., Tufts Medical Center, Boston, MA

I met David Johnson in the fall of 2003, when he arrived from Arkansas for a specialty consultation at our referral center at Tufts Medical Center in Boston. I immediately took a liking to him. How could you not with his down to earth southern manner, and the sense that he represents the soul of the earth? Kind, gentle, but unfortunately very sick. David had a heart disease that he was not responsible in any way for acquiring - he was simply born with a genetic mutation that caused him to develop a cardiovascular condition called hypertrophic cardiomyopathy.

So began a more than 13-year journey with David and his family that I was honored to be part of in helping guide him with expertise and insight about treatment strategies for his heart disease and being honest about what the future may hold for him. They say that the true measure of a person is their ability to go deep and find it within themselves to stand up to adversity…and at the young age of 38 years, David faced life's greatest adversity: his own mortality. His heart was failing, making it increasingly difficult for him to perform even the simplest of daily tasks. Along this most difficult journey, David has fought hard, so hard, and along with his faith and the support of his family, has succeeded in this fight. On May 24th, 2016 David received a new heart at Hershey Medical Center in Pennsylvania.

His story is an amazing one, filled with courage, persistence, and strength, never once losing faith or humility. David's journey out of darkness stands as a testament to others faced with similar dreadful situations of mortality due to a genetic disease like hypertrophic cardiomyopathy. I have no doubt that this work will serve as an inspiration to so many of these patients and their families, filling them with the hope and courage needed to overcome this adversity, to defeat their illness, and have the opportunity to re-engage life with health and happiness.

Martin S. Maron,

Tufts Medical Center

Boston, MA

Prologue

I can see the bathroom door, mid-way down the hall, near the stairs. Trying to ignore the squashed wad of Bubble Yum, black from the foot traffic of a college dorm, I drag myself across the dirty tiles at a snail's pace, weak and slick with sweat, and stinking from the funk of days without a shower. I imagine that I leave a trail of slime behind me as I inch my way down the seemingly endless corridor. I just have to make it to the dorm bathroom before I puke...a lofty goal, though it can't be more than fifty feet from my room.

I should be sitting in music theory class right now, trying not to fall asleep. The class is largely a waste of time because my mind rebels at the thought of dissecting songs like frogs in a high school biology lab. But I'm a struggling first year music major, cowering in the looming shadow of the final, and I'm supposed to be there.

The dorm is a ghost town at 8:45 this Monday morning, except for me, slithering my way toward the community toilets on hands and knees, and eventually my stomach. My gut roils and lurches as I make my way, bit by bit to salvation.

The old asbestos tiles are cold on my bare knees, but I finally make it to a stall and haul myself up with all my strength to hang my head over the toilet. The vomit has no substance because I've not eaten much of anything in two days. I feel like I've run a marathon. When I finally stop retching, I gag a few more times at the thought of being on the floor of a dormitory bathroom. I sag against the toilet, the porcelain cool against my fevered face, and I fall asleep.

The college nurse diagnosed me with Mononucleosis a few days ago; it's been going around. It takes me ten years to realize she's wrong. I'm in heart failure. And I'm slowly dying.

Chapter 1

Rest Assured...

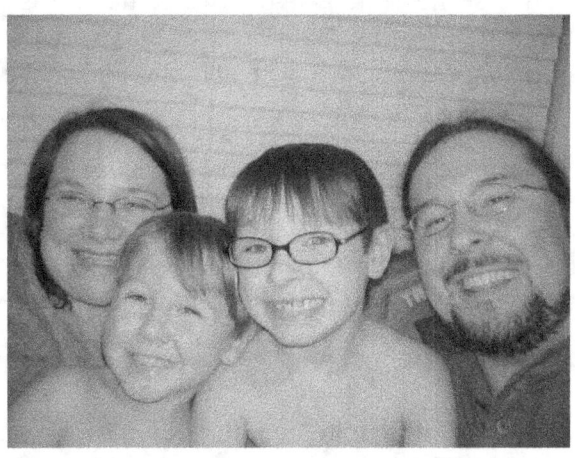

Rest assured – we made our escape
No more suspicion, no more hopeless fate
Pain behind us, look to the dawn
I think we finally found where we belong

To rest our souls, to find a new way
Peace of mind, a brand-new day
Whatever comes our way, it should be easy...

I stare out the window at the subtle golds and sienna's that have crept into the veins of the green leaves these past weeks, a sure sign of approaching autumn and our first Ozark winter. It snows so little in Central Arkansas, and we've been assured by the natives that we'll see plenty here in the northwest corner of the state, a notion that suits the boys just fine. I take a sip of tea and return to the novel I'm writing. Safe at my table in the secluded back corner of the Bentonville library, near the window, where there's enough light to keep me energized, and a wooded view of the backyard to give my eyes a break from the laptop screen.

Snow was one of the big selling points, last year as Rich and I sat at the donut shop by our house in Little Rock, chowing down on his favorite breakfast food – or favorite anytime food. The fall of 2005 seems so long ago now. Brennan was six months old at the time, but at four years, Rich was old and wise enough to understand the big changes we were about to make. We discussed all of it over breakfast that morning.

"So, we would be just like normal people," I said, trying to gauge his reaction.

"You wouldn't be the pastor anymore?" As distracted as he might have seemed by whatever donut he was devouring, I knew he'd never even considered such a thing. I was the Pastor of Calvary Chapel. It's What We Did.

"Nope. We could go to church on Sunday or stay home if we felt like it. And I wouldn't have to leave when we're eating, and I wouldn't be on the phone all the time."

"Would all the people still be mad at you?"

For all my paraphrasing, I remember this question exactly as he said it. It was the crux of the issue really. The reason Christie and I had decided that despite working for a decade to build a ministry that served people we'd loved for nearly fifteen years, it was time to throw in the towel. The preceding year had been a parade of arguments, hostility, passive aggressive anger, abandonment, backstabbing, death and rape threats, nearly being shot once, and counseling everything from incest to domestic violence and sexual assault on a near monthly basis. I could no longer take even a single day away from church business without paying dearly for it upon my return. Calvary Chapel was purposely a refuge for the dysfunctional, the disenfranchised, those on the fringes of the mainstream church; bikers, ex-cons, ex-dealers, ex-whatevers, as well as a handful of folks struggling to escape dangerous or destructive lifestyles. "The Island of Misfit Toys," one member called it.

Problem is, I'm not a misfit. I wasn't raised around drug addiction, alcoholism, divorce, violence, and depression. When I was in junior high, my love of Van Halen and the drums drove me to hang out with the stoner crowd at school, and I'd concluded that these were the "sick" people that Jesus spoke of, in need of a doctor. So, I immersed myself in that culture for nearly twenty years.

But I couldn't do it anymore. They needed a doctor to be sure, but I was not the one for the job. To complicate matters, Brennan, our youngest of two, was extremely ill from a gastrointestinal reaction to penicillin that rendered him unable to process most food. He wasn't thriving or developing properly, Christie hadn't slept more than three consecutive hours in nearly four months, and we'd reached a breaking point. I didn't intend to tell the congregation until the end of January, until I discussed it with some other trusted pastors who were privy to the situation. But subtle preparations for departure meant changes in the way the church functioned, and those were met with a lot of yelling, frustration, and passive aggression that often found a target in both Rich and Brennan, when Christie and I left them in the nursery or the children's church. Rich had witnessed multiple confrontations in the parking lot, outside of my office, in our home, and even in a filled sanctuary.

He also knew Christie and I had been fighting a lot, frustrated, sleep deprived. We hid from him the fact that my assisting pastor and biker friend, Richard, had spent two nights sleeping in his car in our driveway because an ex-member (a cop with a work-related brain injury) had threatened to kill the four of us in our sleep. He'd shown me the service weapon he intended to use the previous week, when I'd talked him into pulling it out of his mouth.

Things were bad, but it had never occurred to Rich that we could just...*leave*.

"We'd live farther away from Gramsy and Pops, and Nana and Pawpaw. About four hours. But we'll visit them a lot, and they can come visit us."

He mulled this over for a few seconds, finished his milk, and shrugged.

"I'd be okay with that."

Leaving that nightmare involved asking permission in many ways. This was self-imposed, to keep from burning bridges with Calvary Chapel and the group of pastors who had supported me for years. But before I even began down that road, Christie and I wanted Rich to be on board. Once he was, I was determined to get out of the volatile situation as quickly as possible.

After the messy business of extracting myself from Calvary Chapel and all things related, we moved to the Ozarks in July of 2006. We found a perfect rental across town from the school where Christie worked toward her associate nursing degree, and ten minutes from an incredible elementary school.

We are happy for the first time in a long time, maybe since Christie and I had married. Brennan and I have a routine; groceries on Monday, the gym on Wednesday. The crown event of them all – Storytime at the library on Tuesday. We fall in love with the kid's librarian who takes a particular shine to Brennan. I've begun my young adult novel and am right at home talking to her about the latest authors and the new Harry Potter book. After, we spend a few hours in the adjacent café, Brennan eating "dinosaur chickens" (Dino chicken nuggets) and watching Sid the Science kid. The café manager gives him full run of the TV, while I study for the few classes I'm taking online. No rush, no hurry, other than to pick up Rich at three, go home and play, eat dinner together, take a walk around the block a few times with our faithful Alaskan Malamute, Nanouq, then stories at bedtime. There's always an Elder Scrolls session on the computer for me before bed while Christie studies. Wash, rinse, repeat. Sounds boring to most people. To me, it's paradise.

On Fridays, Christie has no classes, so I rotate spending the day at Rich's elementary school as the director of the Watch Dog Dads group, or sitting here, at my table in the quiet back corner of the library, working on my novel.

The leaves are changing color, slowly succumbing to the decay that works its damage from within, unaware that at any moment, their summer strength and vibrancy will wane, and they'll fall to the ground, a slow, spiraling tumble, unable to control the winds or seasons that shape their fate.

Chapter 2

Boston (It Only Takes a Day)

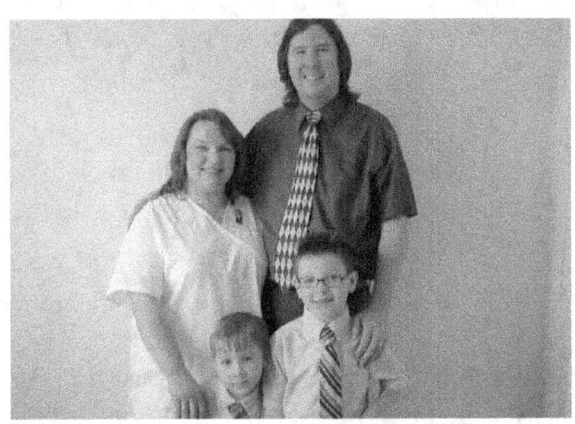

Maybe I'm crazy, maybe I'm wrong,
Maybe there's no reason in the world at all,
Maybe it's random, just the fate of circumstance,
Maybe it's all part of some twisted Master Plan,

What you don't know can hurt you,
What you don't see can bleed you like a dream,

It only takes a day for everything to change,
it only takes a day, it only takes a day,
It only takes a word to blow it all away,
it only takes a day, it only takes a day,

Don't have the time, don't have the guts,
Surely it's mind over matter in the clutch,

Surely panic only feeds my fight or flight,
Surely tears can be held back by shock and spite,

What you don't fear can beat you,
What you don't stand up to can choke you in your sleep,
What you don't face can kill you,
Whatever you flee, will get you in the end,
It only takes a gun to blow it all away,
It only takes a spark to blow up in your face,
It only lets the monster finally have its way,
it only takes a day, it only takes a day

"Well ... you've got a hell of a lot of scarring here." Dr. Maron lays the MRI results on the table between us. "I don't think we can do anything else with meds. I really think it's time to look at transplant."

For the purpose of this book, I wish the conversation had been more dramatic. But it's faithful to Dr. Maron's personality; no sugar-coating, no beating around the bush, no bullshit. The three marks by which I come to judge all other cardiologists.

I think all three of us stop breathing for a few seconds. Christie and I for lack of response, Dr. Maron, waiting for one. My brain finally catches up.

"So, what do we need to do next?" I ask.

"If you lived here, I'd start testing to put you on the transplant list today. I'm worried that even if I were able to, you don't have enough time." He lets that hang in the air, then asks, "Is this the news you were expecting?"

"No," I say. "I was expecting you to tell me I needed a myectomy, but I guess we're way past that point. What's the life expectancy if I actually make it to transplant?" I ask. I already know the answer to this, but I need to hear it from him.

"For men, about five to seven years, average. That's if the transplant takes. The medications are very hard on the rest of the body and complications develop." He seems confused. "Most people have a more emotional reaction," he says. Thinking back on it, I realize he was giving us permission to freak out.

"We don't have time to be emotional," Christie says. "We're only here until tomorrow morning. We need to relocate here, so we need information, and we need to get it right."

No lie, that. We'd flown into Boston the day before and hit the ground running. I'd felt- terrible for six months. My hometown cardiologist thought that being sedentary and near-forty was making me fat. He couldn't find anything wrong, but I knew. Or at least I suspected. Then I'd have a spat of good days and convince myself it was all just in my head. Fearing I'd need a surgery we'd scouted the area before and after my echo and MRI after landing yesterday. We'd told our families that we'd be looking for apartments during our trip; I knew that surgeries involving HCM, my particular heart disease, shouldn't be done just anywhere, and I knew there wasn't a place in Little Rock I'd trust enough anyway, considering my frequent misadventures in various ER's and cardiology clinics over the years. Added to the fact that HCM could be lurking in the genetic makeup of both our boys, we'd been talking pointedly about re-locating somewhere that treated HCM already. I'd spent a few days scouring the internet for apartments and coordinating our schedule, so we could take buses instead of renting a car, which was a challenge, since I couldn't do much walking. We'd missed one of the buses in town and had to walk all the way around the Commons at the hottest part of the day yesterday, and I paid for it last night. HCM has a way of reminding you not to take it lightly. It won't be ignored.

When we'd seen Dr. Maron back in 2003, his entire staff was HCM savvy; receptionists, techs, and nurses. This appointment, in 2010 began differently.

Noreen, the nurse practitioner seemed exasperated that we'd flown all the way from Arkansas, just because I'd gained a lot of weight in my abdomen.

"You're thirty-nine years old, you're more sedentary than you've been in the past. What's your diet like?"

The same uninformed questions and HCM ignorance I'd experienced everywhere else. She checked my ankles for fluid – there was none, of course. HCM causes fluid retention in the abdomen, unlike typical heart failure. Noreen systematically blew off each symptom I complained of. She finished her preliminary exam and left us panicked and frustrated – had we spent all this money and come all this way just have the same argument? It had taken me three months in Arkansas to convince Dr. Allen that something was wrong. Finally, a scope procedure had confirmed "a shadow" he couldn't identify. So here we were.

I hear Dr. Maron's voice in the hall, patiently explaining to Noreen, "… so you won't see any fluid in the ankles, it will be in the abdomen. Look at this…" I assume he's showing her the MRI results I'll see in a few moments. I learn later she's new to the HCM clinic. I write her off as just another unhelpful, uninformed nurse who'll never get it. In the three years that follow, she becomes our family's rescuer, advocate, and a trusted ally. One more person to whom I literally owe my life.

After Dr. Maron drops the bomb, he gives us some more information and tells us to call anytime with more questions. We nearly run out of the clinic, foregoing lunch plans at Legal Seafood around the corner, and opt for a Hertz dealer. No more time for buses. We're headed to Medford to look at as many apartments, schools, and potential nursing jobs as possible before our flight the next day. We're halfway there when we realize we need to eat, though neither of us feel like it. We aimlessly end up at a fast food fish place, a far cry from the crab stuffed flounder and mussels in white wine sauce I'd anticipated on this, my second trip to Boston. I can't think about food.

We debate calling our parents but decide this isn't news I want to deliver over the phone. Christie steps out to call her mom while I wait for the food. I'm sitting in an empty booth doing the math. Five to seven years. Best case scenario, Rich will be seventeen. Still in high school, unmarried. Brennan will just have entered puberty, if that. And this is even if I can somehow miraculously make it to transplant.

Then the nausea comes.

They're calling my receipt number. I choke down the bile. No time for all that right now. We grab the fish, but it sits uneaten between us in the rental as we race for Medford. The only thing I remember about the rest of that day is listening to Christie telling an apartment manager why we were looking and seeing her respond with that look of pity that would become sickeningly familiar within days.

***

Star Wars. I'm one of "those guys." One of my earliest memories is sitting in the backseat of my folk's green Ford station wagon, watching Luke Skywalker, Han Solo, and Princess Leia try to escape the Death Star. When Han Solo (spoiler alert) was frozen in carbonite in The Empire Strikes Back's cliffhanger, my Han action figure promptly went into the freezer. My earliest brush with Schrodinger's Cat – neither alive nor dead, and we wouldn't know until 1983's Return of the Jedi.

In 2018, nearly everyone on the planet is a Star Wars fan. But I'm a Star Wars FAN. Between 1983 and 1999, (the "dark years" as we call them) there were no Star Wars films released, but Del Rey published nearly 90 books, and Dark Horse nearly 200 comic books, continuing the adventures of the main characters, and as many background and minor characters as you could imagine. I own most of them.

When the new Star Wars film was released in 1999, though sickly because of the onset of HCM symptoms, I slept all night on the sidewalk in front of the theater with about fifty other fans to buy early tickets. It was the days before internet ticket purchases, and I considered it worth the health risk. Then I dressed up as a Jedi for opening night. I figure my Star Wars toy and memorabilia collection was at one time worth around $20,000 to the right collector. I own every chronicle of the Clone War conflicts, as well as the fan-assembled military journals and maps. I am fluent in Mando'a (the war language of the Mandalores), Hutteese (both dialects), understand the outer rim trade language of the Jawa's, read Aurebesh (the written form of the "Basic" language in Star Wars), and can recite the history of the Sith with more detail than I can American history. I have no illusions about this being a complete and utter waste of time, but I give myself nerd passion points to assuage the guilt. So yeah, I'm THAT guy.

All this to say, I've taken the message of the Jedi to heart since I was very young. It's been a guiding principle for me, even when I was a Christian pastor. The concept of looking for peace in all situations, staying centered in the midst of chaos, having a larger perspective about my place and context in the universe and in my circle of influence. It's actually a mix Zen Buddhism and mostly Taoist philosophy. I've failed often to maintain that balance of character, but it's served me well when I have. I put a lot of stock in the words that Yoda imparted to Luke Skywalker in 1980's The Empire Strikes Back; "Luminous beings are we," he says, touching Luke's shoulder, "not this crude matter."

But I find little solace in this, or anything else as I keep my nose buried in a Star Wars novel on the plane ride home. Jax Pavan has narrowly escaped Emperor Palpatine's infamous Order 66 (known to the uninitiated as the Great Jedi Purge) and needs passage off Coruscant. A frustrating and dangerous plight, but at least Jax would go down fighting. I wasn't sure whether to fight or curl up into a ball. Either way there would be no escape for me. I trust Dr. Maron implicitly, and if he says it has to be done, that's it.

This is also the first of many times we encounter the inexplicable kindness of strangers. The woman seated next to Christie on the plane offers to let us stay in her in-law quarters if we need to when we come back. It's not an idle offer - she gives us her address and phone number. Bostonians are awesome like that.

Christie and I discuss how to tell my parents, the most difficult conversation we'll have, second only to the kids. They're picking us up from the airport, so we try to plot out the best scenario. I need to talk, so I don't want to drive, but we also don't want to deliver the news while either of them is driving. You never know how someone might react to shocking news. Christie will take the wheel, I'll sit in the back seat. We'll try to make sure Dad's up front with Christie so that I can be in the backseat with my Mom. We hope it's the best way to do it. We're new at this.

They take the news quietly, but with a lot of emotion, particularly once we get back to their house. We can't stay long because we're anxious to see the boys who are with Christie's parents in Searcy, forty-five minutes down the road. We're a bit dismayed to learn later that my folks already knew what was coming because Christie's dad crossed paths with them the day before and mentioned the transplant, not knowing we were waiting to tell them. In retrospect, maybe we should have, but I couldn't bear to do it over the phone.

Throughout this whole mess, we've found that no matter how much you plan and agonize over the right way to do things, whether big or small, something always just gets away from you, slips through the cracks. Just getting the flight back that day makes me realize that even though I don't want to interact with other humans, I have to force my way through the numbness to do it. I'm aware that every relationship I have will now be one-sided. That I'll have to be accommodated, worried about, and eventually unable to reciprocate even the smallest exchanges upon which relationships are built. I can see now that I worried too much about taking care of the needs of others at the beginning – our friends and parents, even accommodating doctors and nurses – to plan for their reactions to our decisions, worrying that we were being inconsiderate, trying not to take advantage of the situation, doing it "wrong." I'm paying for it now, on the other side of the whole thing, all the stuff I held back from people, putting on a brave face so they wouldn't worry or feel awkward. Hiding makes the horror private, and I got trapped with it in my head because I was on eggshells with everyone else's feelings.

Back with the boys after three days in Boston, I grab them up and start tickling them. We roll on the floor, wrestling around and rough-housing. I do a stellar job of hiding the chest pain and breathlessness in the aftermath, but I'm acutely aware that by the time I'm able to do such things again, they'll probably be too big to wrestle with dad. That realization is worse than the conversation about the transplant. If the conversation is hard, the questions that follow the next day, when they've had time to think about the whole business, are brutal.

"Where does the heart come from?"

"Will dad still know us when he has a new heart?"

"Will dad still love the same things he does now?"

"That sounds dangerous. Can people die from heart transplants?"

We've not even broached the subject of having to move away from our Ozark home, their friends, their grandparents, their soccer and skating teams, the library, their homeschool group, their park...

Adults buffer their guilt by telling themselves the lie that children are resilient. They are, but only to a point. We have to - the greater need is often met at their expense. I'm a proud Air Force Brat. My father served his country for over two decades, and I announce that gleefully, every chance I get. I was never active duty myself, but my childhood was shaped by that service, and it's made me who I am more than any other single factor. It's made me resilient, yes, but it's also made me restless, without many lifelong friends, unable to revisit the places where I have so many strong memories, like Italy, Germany, and California. I have no regrets about that – it's more than worth it for the life experience. It didn't leave me psychologically damaged, but it strongly affected my worldview, my perspective on relationships, and my opinions about the influence of culture and environment.

I think the boys are just now, seven years later, starting to realize how this whole thing has shaped and affected them, made them different from their friends. Back then, they looked at the challenges ahead as an adventure. We worked hard to make that so.

Dr. Maron made one thing perfectly clear: I would die if I stayed in Arkansas. My local cardiologist agrees. Transplantation for HCM is so rare, no center in the state will list me. But moving to Boston will strip us of our support system just when we need them most. We designate Boston Plan B.

***

Plan A: find a transplant center within driving distance or move to one close enough to retain our support system. This means not only a med center that knows HCM well enough to keep me alive until transplant but one that can also deal with the sticky problem of listing an HCM patient in the first place. It's going to be an uphill battle, and the odds aren't good.

We're on the phone with Lisa Salberg, the founder of the HCMA, the only patient advocate organization for my disease on the planet. She helped me find Dr. Maron to begin with back in 2003, and she knows more than most general cardiologists about the world of HCM. A center in St. Louis has recently been approved by the organization to treat HCM patients. Transplant may be another thing, but it's worth checking out. St. Louis is six hours away, but way closer than Boston. We make an appointment with both the HCM cardiologist and a transplant doctor. Neither of us want to live in St. Louis, but we make arrangements to see some apartments while we're there. The situation is complicated. Our friends in the Ozarks are great, but the boys aren't comfortable spending three days with any of them, so we either have to drive four hours in the opposite direction to leave them with our parents, or our parents have to come to us. We arrange it and set out for St. Louis.

"You'll never need a transplant," claims Dr. Keith Mankowitz, the "HCM specialist," at St. Mary's Hospital. We've gone to great pains to have my MRI sent from Tufts in Boston. "I don't even need to see it," he says, waving the disk away. "Your ejection fraction is almost normal."

This last statement makes my stomach drop. Without boring everyone to death, let's just say ejection fractions were used to assess patients like me back in the 1980's, before HCM was even labeled correctly. It's only one small piece of the puzzle when it comes to the severity of the disease. We realize we're yet again sitting in a room with a doctor who knows less about the disease than we do. On our way out, I duck into the men's bathroom, sit on the floor, and break down in sobs. This contradiction feels even worse than the initial diagnosis. Who am I to believe? Dr. Maron, obviously. But the temptation to believe Mankowitz is intoxicating. Can I just drive home to the Ozarks and continue on with my life, instead of subjecting myself and my family to this nightmare that's been looming on the horizon ever since we went to Boston a month ago? How are we going to pay for all of this on my meager disability comp and a nurse's salary? It occurs to me, not for the last time, that I may be worth more dead than alive to my family. If I'm gone, so is the problem. Not that I have the guts or courage to do myself in, but I already feel like a walking dead man, not much good for anything to anyone, and more of a burden than a person. No one has made me feel this way. It's just my mind searching for the easiest and quickest escape route. Fight or flight. I don't have much strength to fight.

The following appointment with Dr. Joseph, the transplant cardiologist, goes the other way. She agrees with Dr. Maron and wants to begin testing to get me listed. She's knowledgeable about the disease and understands the urgency of the situation, but Christie has to be at work that night, so we can't stay for any of the testing. We schedule it for the following week.

And so it goes. We make six trips to St. Louis between May and December of 2010. It's a twelve-hour round trip. The boys start going with us and we try to find some fun things to tack on to the end of hospital visits – children's museums, water parks, good restaurants. Back home, we've moved from our perfect little house to a very small apartment in Fayetteville because we can't afford the rent anymore; the trips to St. Louis cost about six-hundred dollars a pop, and the out-of-pocket bills are starting to roll in. Christie can't work much overtime because I'm not able to do as much at home anymore, even on good days. We figure the cramped space is good practice for wherever we'll eventually end up. Our house-hunting in nearby Springdale, Arkansas comes to an abrupt halt. It's self-torture at this point.

The boys complain about none of this – losing their backyard, moving forty-five minutes away from friends, the park, their routine. Having to cram together in a bedroom so small that most of their belongings have to be put in storage. Sitting in waiting rooms for hours while I get tested, the long drives back and forth. Not a peep. I hated it for them. We don't know yet that these are the easy times.

Months roll by. We become increasingly aware that there's some type of contention at St. Mary's between the transplant team and the HCM doc. They don't share information or test results, requiring me to repeat echoes and EKG's back to back several times, all out-of-pocket. By December, I'm still not listed. I've had several sinus infections and problems with restless leg syndrome and need Dr. Joseph to weigh in on safe medications, but it's impossible to communicate with her. It devolves to the point that I'm being given medical advice by the receptionist at the clinic and treated once again like a congestive heart failure patient by the nurses.

The breaking point comes at my last visit with Dr. Joseph, when we ask once again about the plan to navigate the UNOS criteria that I don't meet.

"We'll just have to cross that bridge when we get there," she says, almost confused that I'm concerned about such a thing. In truth, it's almost of more concern than the actual transplant surgery itself. Getting listed initially and moving up that list is everything. As of this writing, twenty-two people die every day on waiting lists for organs. That's nearly eight-thousand people a year. And if my transplant team leader doesn't have a plan, there's an extremely high chance I'm going to be part of that statistic.

"It's going to be tough to actually get you listed because you're a very unique case," she says. "I'm anxious to see what happens. If nothing else, it's going to make for some great research."

As we pull out of the parking lot for the six-hour drive home Christie says, "This isn't going to work. We've got to do something else."

My guts curl up inside me.

"I know."

***

After what has officially been termed, "The St. Louis Debacle of 2010," it makes the most sense to cut to the chase and high-tail it for Boston. And when Christie gets her mind set on doing something, both heaven and hell would have to join forces to stop her. The moment we decide St. Louis is a bust, she becomes single-minded. She spends days online, looking at hospitals, searching job listings, calling, emailing, and trying to find employment there. The 2008-09 school year is overly kind to the medical industry in Boston, as it sees the largest graduating class of nurses in nearly a decade. If it's a blessing for hospitals, who perpetually bemoan the "nursing shortage," it's a curse for any graduating nurse who doesn't have one foot in the door somewhere before the other leaves the commencement podium. All the high-volume medical centers in the greater Boston area find themselves eating their investments in graduates who have to be released from their contracts to pursue work at smaller medical centers. The market is flooded. A majority are currently seeking employment as far away as Rhode Island and northern Maine. There are simply no nursing jobs within a four-hour radius of Tufts Medical Center in Boston, where I need to be listed for transplant; and I'm required to live within that radius.

We hatch Plan C.

While New England hospital budgets restrain them from hiring any more full-time nurses, all hospitals typically get around their staff budgets by hiring temporary nurses – or "travel nurses," as they're called. Companies have sprung up all over the world to facilitate this. They hire and pay the nurses, carry their insurance, and provide furnished housing, while the nurses complete three-month contracts in various locations chosen from a list that the company updates as the contracts become available. Christie sends resumes to several of these, and decides on Cross Country Travel Corp. She is assigned a coordinator, Gale, who provides assignments that meet our criteria, both in terms of Christie's resume and our accommodations. There are no assignments near Boston, but a few close enough to start being seen by Dr. Maron at Tufts on a regular basis. It's all we can do at the moment, with my life-expectancy still unknown.

We'd entertained the idea of travel-nursing as a family around the time Christie graduated the previous year in 2009 and had started homeschooling the boys just to see if we could make it work. Now, we're doing it whether we want to or not. We certainly aren't going to pull them in and out of a new school every three months when contracts change. It isn't a perfect solution, but it's all we can do.

I sit in the floor with Rich as he debates which books to bring. Frannie K. Stein is very popular with both he and Brennan at the moment, but we're emotionally attached to the Nathaniel the Beastologist series. Tough choices. Just like Brennan, we've given him a 6-inch-deep, 20 x 14-inch bin, along with a 4-inch-deep, 10 x 7-inch bin to pack anything he wants to take for the next six, possibly nine months on the road. We've already made room in the van for their extensive Lego collection, some basic kitchen needs, clothes, the Xbox, the geckos, and a few personal things for Christie and myself. My guitar is a must have. It mostly seems like an adventure to the boys, but all I can see is them packing away moments of their childhood and precious keepsakes from grandparents and friends for indefinite storage. How soon before they see that favorite stuffed animal again, or that special coin or knife from Pawpaw? The old P.O. boxes my father painstakingly enclosed and gifted to them are packed and repacked with elaborate care and many tears with their most prized possessions. They're confident they'll be safe there, hidden away with an inscrutable combination lock, kept secret from the world. I take a break from helping with this frequently, excusing myself to take care of some other task, then slipping outside or into the bathroom to take deep breaths and trying to re-center myself. There are kids in more dire circumstances, no doubt; this is a small thing in proportion to the horrors that too many children around the world suffer on a daily basis. The majority of the world's ten-year old's don't have possessions to choose between. But I know this act represents the coming years of their lives in microcosm. They'll be missing their final soccer games, Rich, his final roller-skating competition, and are being asked to leave their first true friends, then the family they'd grown up around. Everything is changing, and not because we're moving to a better life or better job elsewhere. We really don't know what the outcome of all this will be. If it ends badly, I'll have dragged them around the country for nothing, wasting our last time together in a vain attempt to stay alive, a prospect which seems increasingly unlikely.

Rich understands the stakes, but Brennan spends most of these months in bewilderment as our trips to Storytime and the gym abruptly come to an end. There is scarcely time for Christie and me to process it all, and I still wonder what effect our barely concealed fear and anxiety will eventually have on them both.

**

It's not like snow is a big deal in the Ozarks. Unless it's a record snow for that time of year. Unless it's unexpected. Unless it catches even the weathermen by surprise. Unless it falls the night before the big, complicated plan to pack a 26-foot moving van to put all your belongings into storage, move out of an apartment, pack a Honda Odyssey with everything you'll need to live for the next God-knows-how-many years, and drive four hours down a steep mountain in said moving van and Honda Odyssey.

There's no wiggle room. Christie has to be in Hershey, Pennsylvania for orientation in one week.

Plan D: store our belongings in a local storage unit, cram everything else we can in the van, and head down the mountain, hoping for the best. We desperately need our things to be near our families in the Little Rock area – down the mountain – so we can get at them easily during visits home, and so they can mail us anything we might need while abroad. We're moving away from Fayetteville – probably forever. We don't want to leave the majority of our household belongings here for who knows how long. But we have no choice. Christie wades through waist deep snow in the hospital parking lot to get home from her night shift, and the chaos begins.

We reserved a truck, but the U-Haul place is snowed in. We frantically call around until we find someone open and end up with a smaller truck than we need, but the snow has turned us from choosers to beggars, as it were. We call up every person we know in the area to get help with the move, but they're all snowed in. Finally, my writer friend, Tim Koch, shows up with a friend and his son. Between the five of us, we manage to get everything into a storage unit, but not without having to dig the moving truck out of icy ruts a few times. We thank them profusely, then, head back to the apartment, exhausted, to pack the Honda in the dark. After a harrowing trip down the mountain, we arrive at my parent's home in Jacksonville well after midnight.

    We spend a few days with family and friends while tying up loose ends before we set out upon what will become, in retrospect, a trial by fire for our marriage and family. Having conquered the ice and snow, the first of many adversaries to come, we have a few more people to see, a stop or two to visit family in Tennessee, and then we're off on our great adventure.

Chapter 3

Over the Brink

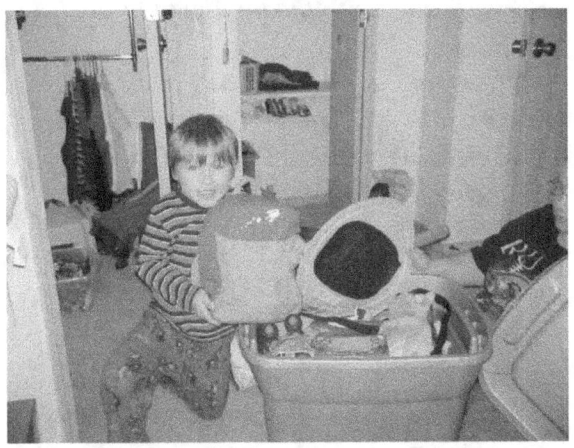

It always sneaks up from behind, like,
hey brother - think you could spare me a life,
The scale is tipped, the kung-fu grip,
caught me in the blind – hoodwinked,

Somebody's knocking down my door,
I'm lying, face down on the floor,
Downward spiral, failed revival, happens in the blink,
I was just fine all of this time, now we're headed to the brink,

I can't seem to dig my heels in,
pay for the time that I've been stealing,

Conversations from Room 1170

Simon says at gunpoint, there's no use this is the new joint,
Over the brink, Over the brink

Dead weight, I'll just tote around,
Sleep deprivation, the newest pill in town,
Stop the clock, the chopping block,
flailing, sinking, drowning in the drink,
I can't tread water all my lowlife,
Lurking, cower in the half light,
One percenter, I'm a winner, flash the plastic crown,
Tires squealing crank the sound,
we're speeding with the top down to the brink,

Drugs and daggers are my trademark,
the bullet's riddled with my teeth marks,
Fetch the axman, it's the Pressing,
spite and honor, all that I bring,
Over the brink, over the brink

And every day, just pulls-me-down,
all I ever, hear-the- sound of-
Best laid plans, crash to-the-ground,
one more test, look what-we've-found

It started with the fish.

I mean, not really, but I think the fish was the first time in years that I was reminded that something was very wrong. I already knew I was sick. That bomb had been dropped back in 1998, after speculation of lung disease, stomach cancer, or possibly even HIV, until a cardiologist finally diagnosed me with Hypertrophic Cardiomyopathy – the same disease that sneaks up on athletes and causes sudden cardiac death. I was incredibly active at the time. It was pre-parenthood, and we not only owned a floor and marble servicing company that I'd built from the ground up, I was moonlighting as a drummer in a three-piece hard rock band, fronting my own pop band, and sitting in with numerous other projects. All this while being the worship leader and assistant pastor of a local Calvary Chapel. At first, I was told I was at risk for the dreaded Sudden Death thing and had only months to live. This prompted a messy sale of the business for much less than it was worth and moving almost two hours away from our lives to live with Christie's parents for nearly a year. All of my activities stopped, and Christie hastily found a job. Our finances were in ruins, and with our pathetic self-employed insurance, my medications cost nearly $1100 a month. We lost the house we were living in with the intent to buy, and nearly had our car repossessed. I eventually had to quit my work with the church.

But I didn't die within months. With help from Dr. Van De Bruyn, a local cardiologist, and our parents, we slowly pulled ourselves out of the pit, moved back toward Little Rock and the church. The pastor was eventually fired, and I ended up with the responsibility, if not the authority. I was walking around expecting to drop dead at any moment, and I lived like it. Carpe Morbidis! as it were. I eventually started singing with some musician friends in a local cover band on and off for extra cash while I was a pastor, while bands I would have played for went on to win Grammy and American Music awards, and record gold and platinum selling albums. But I continued to write songs; I have always written songs – I can't stop really. I can see a bottle cap lying in a parking lot and it sparks an idea for a song. I tried to adjust to the idea that the course of my life had changed forever – that I would never have a career in music, and any connection I had to that "right place/right time" world had disappeared with my health. Though I eventually found other meaningful pursuits, such as writing, game design, and cooking, I don't know that I'll ever fully be at peace with having that dream snatched away the moment it was at my fingertips.

Then my original visit to Boston in 2003, and Dr. Maron. In retrospect, Dr. Maron seems obvious to this story. He would become, to my mind, a towering figure; part-time counselor, full-time anchor, the man who saved my life without touching a scalpel. That's his job, of course, but he went far beyond it multiple times.

Mindi Barger, however unintentionally, saved my life as well. She came into our lives one Sunday morning after church in the spring of 2003. A friend of our worship leader's family, she reluctantly came to see what Calvary Chapel was all about. When we were introduced she mentioned that she also had a heart disease, called HCM. Her mother suffered sudden cardiac death at a young age, her older sister had been transplanted, and she had another sister and brother with the same heart disease – that second sister has been transplanted as well since then. After trading symptom stories, as we chronically ill people tend to do, she concluded that I also had HCM.

"Nah. Mine's called Hyper.... something. Hypertrophic Cardiomyopathy."

"Right, HCM," she said.

"No, it's like a thickening of the heart muscle, sometimes it can obstruct blood flow…"

Mindi over enunciated each word as if talking to a child. "Hypertrophic. Cardio. Myopathy. HCM."

We raced home from church and jumped online. Why would I expect to find anything? I'd been scouring the web for years looking for info on Cardiomyopathy but there was never a mention of the Hypertrophic part, or anything related much to my particular condition. But a Google search for "HCM" rewarded us with a windfall of articles, medical journal entries, and most importantly, the link to a patient advocate website called the HCMA. It was a lifeline to a woman named Lisa Salberg.

I called first thing Monday morning to be greeted by a sassy, unapologetic non-Christian lady with a Jersey accent. Lisa Salberg entered my life that day and ends up also saving it on three different occasions to date. I owe more to this trio – Dr. Maron, Mindi Barger, and Lisa Salberg – than I'll ever be able to express or repay. If not for them, I wouldn't be telling you this story. There would be no story to tell. I'd have probably died at the age of thirty, leaving behind my wife, a three-year-old Richard, and the thrilling tale with which I'm regaling you would never have taken place.

"Go to Boston," she told me, after I'd unraveled the rambling story of my diagnosis. "See Dr. Marty Maron. He runs the HCM clinic there."

My mind boggled. A hospital with a whole clinic devoted the HCM? I couldn't even find a cardiologist in Arkansas who knew what the hell the disease even was, or how to treat it.

So, in April of 2003, we went. Dr. Maron informed me that not only was I not at risk for sudden death, I was being over-medicated, and the side-effects were probably worse than the actual disease. Dr. Maron's insight sustained me for six more years. In 2005 we left the ministry, and for all intents and purposes, our affiliation with church and organized Christianity (which is an even more complicated story than this one, chronicled in my album "Instead of Wither"). We moved to the Ozarks and learned what it was to be happy. Christie fulfilled her lifelong dream of becoming a nurse, urged on by the dearth of knowledge about my heart disease in Arkansas. I convinced myself that I would be one of those many people who lived a long, full life, medicated to suppress the symptoms of HCM. I was limited, but we all adjusted. Christie graduated to work at a local hospital in 2009. The boys played soccer. We made friends. I started writing a book. We began establishing roots.

But HCM lurked. On any given day, it can progress, for unknown reasons, causing loss of heart function. Over time, the heart muscle becomes stiff and inflexible, causing a host of other problems. Because part of the heart muscle becomes so rigid, the remaining healthy muscle has to carry the load of the dead weight.

But just as the disease can progress for reasons unknown, it can also plateau unexpectedly, leaving the heart diminished, but still functioning, at least the part that hasn't become stiff and inflexible. It's impossible to know when this downward spiral will continue, when the next stair step will be. Days? Months? Years? It's difficult to plan very far ahead, but when your health changes so randomly, all you can really do is adapt and hang on.

***

The problem isn't so much that HCM is a rare disease. We know that roughly 1 in every 500 people carry the gene. Not all are symptomatic, and some will never even know they have it. A smaller group actually suffer from fatigue, shortness of breath, chest pain, arrhythmias, and other debilitating effects. Fewer still ever progress to the point of needing transplant. So few, in fact, that back in 2011, there were no actual protocols for listing an HCM patient for transplant. HCM patients simply didn't and couldn't meet the criteria called for by the Organ Procurement/Transplant Network (often called OPTN or UNOS). It was designed decades ago for patients with Congestive Heart Failure, the most common problem requiring transplant. The criteria called for patients to be in such bad shape that they needed continuous IV drips of dopamine and dobutamine (known as inotropes) to treat heart failure, and be admitted to the hospital, usually full time, with some type of assist device, like a pacemaker or defibrillator or an LVAD. I'm oversimplifying here for the sake of brevity. Let's just say it was complicated.

    Inotropes are contra-indicated for HCM patients, meaning, at best, they do nothing to help, and at worst, they can actually make some patients feel sicker in higher doses. Pacemakers and defibrillators can help some HCMers, but when the heart becomes as enlarged as mine was, the only solution is transplantation. There's no point in being admitted to a hospital, since there are no devices or medication drips to monitor. Which means even if a patient manages to get listed, there's the additional problem of accumulating hospital admission time - the largest factor at play in terms of moving up the waiting list. No hospital admission time, no "accumulated hours" on the waiting list.

Transplant is an extreme measure for HCM, so rare in fact, that in early editions of the HCM handbook used by most professionals (and written by Dr. Maron's father, Dr. Barry Maron), transplant warranted only a single sentence. So OPTN saw no point in writing exceptions into the protocols for HCM patients. At the time of this writing, these criteria are changing to better accommodate people like me, due in large part to Lisa Salberg of the HCMA, and Dr. Maron, as well as my particular case. But back then, all of this created a spider's web of red tape for both the cardiologists and the patient.

HCM is also sneaky. Unpredictable, inscrutable too. Most HCM literature mentions the risk of sudden death, but that's not as much of a danger now that we know more about the disease. The solution usually involves medications and, in the case of patients who are truly at risk for sudden death, implantable devices such as defibrillators or pacemakers. Devices shock the heart back into a normal rhythm before anything really bad happens. In worst case scenarios, heart surgeons perform a myomectomy or septal ablation in which they literally cut or burn away some of the stiffened heart tissue to prevent blockages in the heart and make its job easier. Any of these methods can typically "fix" the HCM symptoms enough that the HCMer can live a normal, if less physically active life (one without competitive sports, for starters). Because the heart is so labored, most HCM patients become hyper-attuned to the smallest shifts in their health. Increased heart rate, slight dehydration, digestion, and even slight changes in sleep patterns or weight gain and loss.

Which brings me back to the fish.

I'd battled with HCM for years and it had already put me through the ringer. But the fish was the exact "uh-oh" moment in that downward spiral. Christie had taken the kids somewhere for the weekend and left me at home to finish up a draft for my novel, The Ghost of Maddingbrew. I didn't want to lose any time cooking for just myself, so I picked up a few of those TV dinners - not the microwave ones, the kind you put in the oven. I'd been eating really healthy - homemade fruit juice, yogurt, and lots of raw veggies - and working out several times a week. But the TV dinners were a quick, albeit nasty solution to my time crunch.

After eating the first sodium-laden fish dinner, I sat at the computer unable to work. Waves of nausea swept over me unlike anything I'd experienced before. I thought it was food poisoning, but as the night went on, I realized the pain was coming from my chest, not my stomach. It's tempting to think my body was reacting to the faux-food, but it's clear to me now that the HCM simply chose that moment in time to progress again. Salt, stress, trans-fatty acids, lack of exercise - HCM doesn't necessarily get worse because of these things, though it can certainly make the symptoms much worse. Adding a lot of salt to HCM can lead to fluid overload and flash pulmonary edema (a risk even without a high-salt diet). Mostly, HCM keeps its own schedule and can't be hurried along or held back by much of anything external. It's a hard concept to get our heads around, living in a society where we're told that Oreos cause heart attacks and Kale is the key to eternal youth. HCM doesn't abide by the rules of diet and exercise. It's in control, and there's nothing that can be done to wrest that control from it. We can only react and respond.

My sleeping changed. I couldn't get comfortable in bed, tossing, turning, feeling like I'd eaten too much too late. I looked under the covers for some reason one morning and noticed my stomach bulging. I jumped up and weighed myself in the bathroom, something I did from time to time, but having been skinny my whole life, it wasn't habit. I knew I'd been hovering between 175 and 180 for years. That morning the scales report a whopping 205. I turned sideways to the mirror. Where did the beer belly come from? I didn't even drink beer; I'm a wine guy. Or in a pinch, trough water or lamp oil. Anything but beer. Maybe I wasn't exercising enough? It was all fluid retention, though I didn't understand the full implications yet.

But just like you can't make HCM better with exercise or rest, you can't make it worse with fried fish and beer. So really, the fish had nothing to do with it. It was just the moment I knew. I knew my perfect, ordered world, for which we'd fought so hard and endured so much, was going to crumble around us. Before the tests and the poking and prodding began. I just knew.

Over the following weeks, I became unsettled, irritable, and felt frail all the time. I had searing pain in my lower back - so bad that Christie had to come home to help me get up from my desk chair one day. In actuality, my liver and kidneys were struggling to deal with the massive amount of fluid I was retaining. It's one of the first things that happens when HCM progresses. There's risk of flash-pulmonary edema - drowning in your own fluids. In the ER, there is the danger of being given too much fluid or too much diuretic, which can dramatically affect the patient's vascular system, causing immediate and lasting deadness.

Finally, Dr. Allen, agreed to perform an echocardiogram ahead of schedule, after the holidays and found what he called "a shadow." That was 2010, a year that will forever live in infamy in our family. The year started with an impromptu trip to North Carolina to help our niece who was in a dire domestic situation. The trip was expensive, and I was feeling worse and worse. We returned the following week and within days suffered the loss of a beloved great uncle on Christie's side of the family. I awoke a few mornings later to find Nanouq lying in a puddle of her own urine, unable to walk. The vet called it cancer. Something had erupted and caused a brief paralysis. She needed surgery, but she wouldn't survive it. We said goodbye and I spent the next few weeks in a state of abject loss. I'd trained her as a utility dog from a puppy. She went everywhere with us and had weathered the storm of my initial diagnosis faithfully. Even with all that was to come, I was in a fog for months, trying to understand how she could be gone so quickly, with so little warning. I've had trouble connecting with a dog on any level since her. I hope I will someday.

It was in this state of shock, loss and financial stress that I underwent my echocardiogram and scope in February of 2010. The "shadow" prompted closer investigation, so Dr. Allen scoped me (a TEE – transesophageal echo) to get a better look. I vaguely remember his worried expression as I awoke from the sedation.

"You were right. Something's going on. I think you need to go see your guy in Boston."

So, Christie and I found ourselves back there, seven years after the initial trip, on our eighteenth wedding anniversary for a new echocardiogram, stress test, EKG, and most importantly an MRI. I figured there was a surgery or procedure in my future, probably a myectomy. Something fairly straightforward and very low risk, possibly something that could even be done back in the Little Rock area.

This was all very House, right? Everyone thinks their medical problem is unique. I had a lot of difficulty accepting just how rare my condition was. I didn't even fit in with the HCM community, a community that identifies itself partly by the obscurity of its disease. I started to loathe the word "unique."

The other bullet ricocheting around the room was the uncertainty of the next progression. By the time we gave up on St. Louis, I'd survived longer than the six months Dr. Maron projected. All I knew is that when I had the really bad days, I felt like I was going to die right then.

Dr. Maron warned us that day in 2010 that a transplant was not the cure all it sounded like. I knew it wouldn't be like on TV, but it only took a few days to realize the world of transplants, with its lists, criteria, statuses, regions, and protocols was far more complicated than any television drama could ever faithfully portray.

Chapter 4

On the Lam

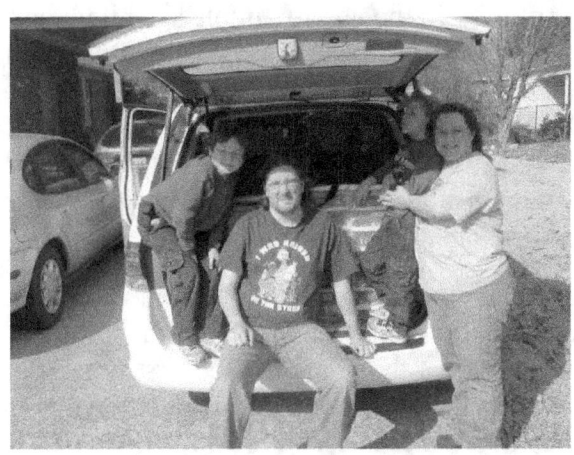

All we own, sitting on our back,
Fear in tow, speeding down the blacktop,
All we know, disappear behind us,
Through ice and snow, never to return,

Start it up, we've gotta move,
Everywhere we roam, nowhere we choose,
Burn it down, there's nothing left to lose - we're on the lam

Parts unknown, here there be monsters,
Off the road, into the wild,
Broken down, we stumble through the forest,
Lost in the dark and the wolves are closing in,

Fall on the mercy, the kindness of strangers,
Grace for fair-weather friends who could only talk the talk,

Clinging tight to the solace of each other,
Walk if you can't run, crawl if you can't walk...
(and when you can't to that...well, you know the rest...)

Resolved but anxious, we wait for our food to come. Agradocio's Italian restaurant in Harrisonburg, Virginia, a little joint in the strip mall across from the hotel. We're one of two families in the whole place, so it's quiet and cozy, a fire crackling softly in the nearby fireplace while Frank and Dean serenade us from the overhead radio. We're still pre-smartphone in 2011, and just getting acquainted with our cantankerous dashboard GPS. I know nothing of Yelp or Hotels.com, and in the true tradition of Christie's father, we'd set out that morning from my Aunt Vicky's house in Dickson, Tennessee with no hotel reservations or dinner destination.

The boys are tired but swept up in the excitement and trepidation of the new and unknown. Christie and I don't say much, lost in our own thoughts. It's the first time in our married lives we're well and truly out of reach of anything familiar; family, friends, landscape. I take as deep a breath as I'm able. I don't know it yet, but I'm starting to finally shed the skin I've worn for so many years, the weight of dropped baggage from the last two decades slowly falling away. Here, in this place, where no one knows me but the three people at the table, I'm no longer Pastor Dave, or the front man for The Dreadnaughts, nor the drummer for Ground Zero, the leader of the Watch Dog Dads organization, the owner of Picture Perfect Floor Care, or the guy who "knows" some of those rock stars. I'm just a husband and father, a guy with a heart problem who loves music and books. I'd decided in the Ozarks it was more than I ever needed to begin with, but here, in this place, at this time, finally, no one expects me to be anything more. I have no reputation, no image, no expectations to meet, and I'm free to think as I want, to speak my mind, and not be judged by anyone based on who they think I am because of who I have been. It's terrifying and intoxicating.

We all understand, even Brennan at the age of six, that this moment marks the beginning of a difficult and treacherous road. That much has been asked, and even more will be demanded of us from both our situation and one another. There's no need for some formal lecturing or parental decree of expectations. We've all chosen to do this together, and to do it to the end, whatever that means. Since this began last spring, we've been living by the "old saying" (adapted from Martin Luther King Jr.) that Mal and Zoe quote to a broken-down war-buddy in an episode of the TV series, Firefly: "When you can't run, you walk, when you can't walk, you crawl. And when you can't crawl, well...then you get someone to carry you." We've taken many of Joss Whedon's lessons from that show to heart, but that admonition from Dr. King will come to play a more vital role in our survival and sanity than we can guess at this, our inaugural meal.

Our port of destination: Hershey, Pennsylvania, Penn State Medical Center. We will be there two days later, hopefully sitting in a clean, furnished apartment, Christie with a three-month job awaiting the following week. We've made a list of things we'll need to buy immediately: toiletries, shower curtain, kitchen and cleaning items, and a grocery list to get us through the first few days, avoiding the expense of eating out again after being on the road.

***

It's a good thing Pennsylvania turns out to be relatively easy, both for Christie at work, and for the boys and me, but it spoils us a bit. The apartment is nice, convenient to everything we need, and close to the hospital. Nearby Lancaster, Philadelphia, the Poconos, and other more local libraries, restaurants, and historical sites keep us busy, and homeschooling is more hands-on than ever. I wonder how we would have altered our plan had it been any other way - future assignments will not be so comfortable.

Christie makes things happen. Once she puts her mind to it, no matter how boring or difficult, it's going down. Despite her inherent courage and confidence, she loathes change, and so spends the night before she starts each new contract curled around the toilet, throwing up her toenails. She's a lot like her father, Layton, who's still irritated that he can't use his dial phone and maintains a deep suspicion of computers because of a bad experience with one in the late 70's. A new job is a huge disruption of her world – as a nurse, she wants to be tight with the rest of her team and know that they have one another's backs. Unfortunately, travel nurses are often held at arm's length by the others, regarded as uncommitted and unconcerned. They get saddled with the most difficult patients and the dirtiest work. This was the case for Christie, but at each new assignment, she proved herself quickly, and by the time her twelve weeks were up, she was usually offered a full-time position. She always declined; we had to get to Boston.

I hook up with the local homeschool co-op and the boys look forward to swimming at the YMCA on cold Fridays and running around at the park with the group during the warm ones. Field trips, activities, new friendships, the dairy farms, the rolling hills and friendly people make Pennsylvania easy to love. Through a series of mishaps and inexperience, our next assignment is a three-month contract in the half-a-horse town of Danville, about two hours north.

Geisinger Hospital in Danville services a huge portion of rural Central Pennsylvania. Farmers, Amish, coal-miners, and small-town country folk living in this-or-that-burg/ville/ton. Most "towns" are little more than thirty houses clustered around a gas station, grocery store, and a dying downtown area replete with mid-19th century churches and libraries. Danville could be a template for this part of the country, though a bit more trafficked because of the medical center, which is clearly the only thing propping up the town's otherwise stymied economy.

Travel Nursing companies respond eagerly to Geisinger's call for staff that summer, resulting in a disastrous nurse-to-housing ratio. There simply aren't enough apartment buildings in Danville to house everyone, so Christie's company resorts to house rentals. Some nurses are being paid mileage to drive in from over an hour away. We're more complicated because we travel as a family of four, and Christie insists that the company find housing on the first floor unless there's an elevator. Stairs make my heart rate jump so high my eyeballs nearly pop out. Too many times up and down and I'm out of commission for days.

We arrive at the address given by Christie's coordinator to find a decrepit two-story home, settled about fifteen minutes outside of Danville in Washingtonville (why not Washingtonvilleburgtown?" my mom and I often ponder). We slowly realize Danville must seem a metropolis to the population of Washingtonville. Ours is one of about twenty residences, along with a single pump gas station and a grocery store featuring dust-covered items so far past the expiration date it's difficult to make out the original color of the packaging.

Christie is devastated. Our rooms are on the second floor, the water smells and tastes of sulfur and chlorine, and the living room is so tiny that all four of us can't fit into it at once. There's no evident internet connection or air conditioning, and the furniture is salvaged from cheap hotels, complete with tube television bolted to the huge cabinets that take up a fourth of the already cramped rooms.

"What have I done?" she whispers tearfully that night. "What have I gotten us into?"

"We'll make it. It's not that bad," I say.

"How is it not that bad?" she asks. "It's horrible…"

"The boys are fine. I'll be fine."

This is my first Livestock and Breakables moment that I can recall. I've been jotting notes down for a potential song about how even though sometimes things aren't your fault, they still happen because of you. I have no working title yet, but the lines go in my notebook for later:

*"Did you drop it on the floor?
And they told you where it came from there's no more?
Did the pieces cut you when you tried
to sweep them off the ground,
And they told you what was lost cannot be found?"*

What if it was going to be like this from now on? How could we turn back, even if we wanted to? It feels like a bait and switch, the opposite experience from the last three months in Hershey.

The boys, becoming more accustomed to these ever-shifting conditions, are fine. I was too, for about the first month. As the days grew hotter, the paltry window unit we'd coerced out of the landlord leaves me in a perpetual sweat. My attempts at cooking in the tiny kitchen, with no countertops and burners that continually smoked, are frustrated at every turn, resulting in many meals eaten at either the Chinese or pizza place - Washingtonville is too far removed from civilization for delivery of any kind. I'm surprised FedEx runs here. The internet is too slow for more than two devices to be connected to it – service drops repeatedly. Worst of all, we are in a cellular dead-zone, cutting us off from communication with Christie while she works night shift in town. Even switching over to smart phones with a local service doesn't help.

Washingtonville sits in the shadow of a coal processing plant which, according to the tour we took in desperation for something to do, doesn't create any pollution due to some fancy filter system they voluntarily installed. Yet the smokestacks, clearly visible from our bedroom window, belch out white smoke all hours of the day and night. I'm having more chest pain than ever. Is it my heart or the smoke?

***

It's been a long week, and at the end of it, the first of many dire warnings of what's to come. Gettysburg is on our list of places to visit, corresponding with the boy's study of the Civil War, so we spend two days there and by the time we reach the memorial museum, I can barely make it from one exhibit to the next without having to sit down somewhere.

My parents are passing through Hershey on the way to visit friends in northern PA, so we meet them for lunch on the way back and invite our homeschool friends, the Folsons. We're eating ice cream at a sidewalk café in the afternoon when my cell rings. It's Dr. Kiernan, the transplant guy from Tufts.

"We got the labs back. Everything looks good for now."

"What was the blood type?" Something you'd think I'd already know, but labs and blood draws aren't figuring into the equation very heavily at this point.

His hesitation tells me all I need to know. "O positive."

My stomach turns. Yet another imperative transplant detail that TV shows and movies manage to gloss over. Arguably the very most important detail. In 2011, an O+ blood type for an HCM patient in burn-out seems like a passive death sentence. While an O+ donor heart can be implanted in anyone without fear of antibody conflicts, recipients with an O+ blood type can only receive an O+ heart. In other words, even if I'm the only transplant candidate with an O+ blood type on the entire waiting list of about 4,000 people in my region, I will be passed over every time for every other blood type that's higher on the list than me, though some likely in less urgent need than I. This means everyone on the list competes only with others of the same blood type. O+ blood types are competing with everyone. Added to the fact that my HCM keeps me from meeting several other criteria on the list, and the fact that I'm taller than average, the prognosis is extremely grim.

Christie and I do a terrible job hiding our disappointment and dread as we relate the bad news to the Folsons and my parents. They turn the conversation to something else pretty quickly, and I don't think they can really be expected to understand the implications of the news. I've found this to be common with friends and family all along this journey; it's got to be difficult to absorb how precarious the whole situation is, how even seemingly small details related in a single phone call can be a matter of life or death; it's hard for us to grasp at times. From the outside, I'm sure it just seems like medical complications that the doctor can fix, whereas transplant candidates quickly start crunching numbers. It's like trying to buy tickets to a one-time, sold-out performance. There's a limited number of seats; you either get one or you don't. Doctors can't convince UNOS to change the rules because the patient will die. Twenty-two families learn that cold, hard fact every single day in the United States. It's difficult to receive news like this and just carry on with your day, eating ice cream, making small talk, trying to pretend you weren't just told you're going to die. You have to keep living while you can.

My folks are gracious enough about our living situation, but it's late, so they head back to the hotel. Finally, after the long week, I'm alone with my boys. Looking forward to a clean (though chlorinated) shower and picking up our nightly reading of Harry Potter, I sit down at the desk in the living room to take my shoes off.

I've been nauseous all day, but now a wave sweeps over me so forcefully that I taste bile in my throat, and I clutch the back of the chair with both hands to keep from falling over. My heart feels like it's lurching back and forth, up and down in my chest, and a pain shoots all the way down my left arm. Heart attack? "What an awful place to die," I think. I always knew this might happen, and between attempts not to pass out, I curse myself because the boys are going to be the ones to find me. Just the cherry on the poop sundae of the last year in their lives.

The astounding thing about this whole story, this journey (at least to me) is the way Rich has handled the whole thing, this incident being the first emergent of many to come. He's eleven years old but doesn't panic. I've never known him to. He helps me get my shoe back on, and grabs my cell phone, telling Brennan to get dressed again because we're going to the hospital. We've never had to do this that he can remember, but he takes over like an experienced EMT, prioritizing and delegating. It's only then I truly realize the danger of Washingtonville's tech vortex. There is no cell service, and there's no landline, owing to the three-month rental to Christie's company. Rich tries to call Christie, but of course, the call won't go through. He tries 911. Call can't be completed. The Public Enemy song, "911 is a Joke," starts playing in my head and I try to appreciate the irony of this being the last song I'll ever hear. If I'm going out, not much better way to do it than with Chuck D. and Flavor Flav as the soundtrack.

There's no chance of contacting Christie, but I remember my parents have iPhones. We're still in the flip phone stage, but with Rich's help, I get turned around in the desk chair and boot up the computer. My chest is starting to hurt badly, and breathing is a challenge. I can't panic in front of the kids. Brennan makes quick work of packing an overnight bag, just in case, and I open Skype. I've never made a computer-to-cell call before, but our old friend and housemate, Robin Walters, used to Skype with her boyfriend (now husband) Joe this way and I remember her telling me about it a few years back. Rich runs to see if Mike, the downstairs neighbor is home. Looks like I have to deposit money into my Skype account. I go through that process using PayPal, passwords and all. Time crawls as my heart races even harder in its helter-skelter rhythm.

Please work, please work.

Rich bounds back up the stairs and shakes his head. No Mike. But Skype is ringing.

I nearly pass out from relief when mom answers. Within fifteen minutes she's racing us all to the hospital. Once the cell phone is in range, I tell Christie to meet us in the ER.

It's atrial fibrillation – A-fib, the despised enemy of HCM patients. Essentially, the structural corruption of the heart tissue causes short-circuits in the heart's electrical system, which in turn make it jump out of rhythm. It rarely returns to normal sinus rhythm on its own. This is a new problem – and pointed message that the disease is progressing again, at least in the electrical department.

My folks take the kids back to the hotel while Christie and I spend a long night in the ER, me on a beta-blocker drip which we doubt will help. The ER docs seem to know HCM pretty well, the first time that's ever happened to us, and graciously call Tufts to get instructions for how to proceed in my case. If the medication doesn't work, I'll have to be cardioverted – shocked, as in "1, 2, 3, CLEAR!" – back into sinus rhythm. Tufts says it's safe, but I'm unsettled, knowing how often I've been the exception to the rule. We have to wait eight hours since I've recently eaten, so we settle in for another five. Was it the stress and exhaustion of the last week that caused this? Or just another random symptom of HCM, rearing its head without cause or explanation?

When the time comes, they sedate me, Christie holding my hand. I don't remember falling asleep, but I come back to the world through a brilliant neon flash and whirlwind of kaleidoscopic colors that reminds me of a Yes album cover. I want to stay, but then the overhead lights and the voices of the nurses are upon me again, and I feel my chest burning - but I can breathe again. The doctor looks a bit shaken, as does Christie.

"We had to hit you twice," she says. "Get to your guy in Boston and see an electrophysiologist. This won't be the last time this happens."

Great.

***

I sit in the stairwell, crying as I squeeze my left arm hard into my chest. The boys have gone to sleep, following Harry Potter (which they never quite seem to fall in love with the way that I have). With each passing day, the pressure becomes more intense. I suspect that it's the air in Washingtonville(burgtown), but I'm on all the medication I can tolerate.

My parents left after the night of A-fib and Christie had to work. I wasn't supposed to drive so it was the weekend before we could get smart phones. We were all holding our breath until then, but they can't get reception either. Our nerves are wrecked until we finish the assignment a few weeks later, hoping against hope the A-Fib stays its hand until we can get back to civilization.

It has been a particularly bad day. We spend most of Christie's down time back in the Hershey area with the Folsons, who are becoming close friends. Rich is in the middle of hockey season when we take the Danville assignment, but it's close enough we can make the drive back on Saturdays. The Folsons graciously offer their guest room so we can come down for INCH park days on Fridays, stay for hockey, and return on Sunday. At the Folsons, we talk, play games, eat out, and discover all the fun things to do in central Pennsylvania. Christie is tired most of the time because this leaves us little time to just vegetate, but we figure this is a temporary thing – we leave in August for a new assignment – so we have fun while we can. It's a much-needed reprieve from the weight and worry of the last year and the little apartment in Washingtonvilleburgtown is depressing and boring.

But this particular day, the last of several spent in Hershey with the Folsons, I'm in agony. We eat at Red Robin that night, and I draw into myself, drowning in a sea of people and voices. The chest pain is so intense I can't pay attention to the conversation, and I don't eat much. Everyone is so loud, so crammed together, and I endure the meal in a trance-like state, that hopefully goes unnoticed by Christie or the Folsons, because of the noise and buzzing activity around us.

We drive home so Christie can work, but once I'm alone, I can't hold back the tears anymore. The pain is so intense, and the gravity of our situation hits me particularly hard this night. We've been on the road for half a year, and we're no closer to Boston than when we set out. Tufts wants to list me, but we're outside of the four-hour window required for me to be listed. The disease has stopped progressing for the moment, but the symptoms leave me more diminished every day, and there's always the fear of the A-fib coming back. Winter is coming, and we decide to take an assignment back in Little Rock to end the year. Holidays with our families, probably for the last time. When we head back north, we know it will be to stay.

***

Fall and the holidays of 2011 pass amidst meet-ups with old friends, and a few trips back to Bentonville, where we visit the library and Rich's old elementary school. Time has moved on and there's not much that connects us to Little Rock or Bentonville anymore except our families and a few friends we've stayed current with via Facebook.

We're at my brother Darrell's house in Sherwood, to celebrate a birthday (as usual, I don't remember who's…) and it's the first time we've seen several people since my transplant news. As much as I enjoy performing and public speaking, I'm usually ill at ease in small groups. I feel awkward, make too many jokes, and inadvertently draw unwanted attention to myself. This has gotten worse now that I'm headed for a heart transplant. It's all anyone wants to talk about, and all other aspects of our life tend to fade into the background. It's no one's fault but I become quickly exhausted explaining the tangled mess we're in with UNOS and the rarity of my disease, and especially the need to be transplanted for it. It's complicated to explain, hard to condense, and so much has happened that the story is cumbersome. I meander a lot between the pool where the boys are playing and into the air conditioning where everyone else is eating and chatting.

There's no exact trigger I can remember, but I suddenly break out in a cold sweat, and my forehead feels incredibly hot, like a flash fever. It feels like the walls are closing in, and all I can hear are the echo of voices. Fight or flight overtakes me more intensely than I ever knew was possible. I've been frightened and in mortal danger several times during my years in the ministry, but this doesn't compare. Not even close. Am I having a heart attack?

When I was in fourth grade, I stumbled upon a teenager shooting heroin in the quiet of the large woods near my house. He chased me, but I was able to make it to my bike and outpace him to the street before he could catch up. I don't know why he chased me, but it was the most terrifying experience of my childhood. In my early thirties, while in ministry, a man pointed a pistol at my face, when I invaded the crash/crack-house where he was sleeping it off to get his young nephew out of the dangerous environment. I de-escalated the situation and the man let us leave, but I was at gunpoint until we cleared the hall, two rooms, and the front door. Another time, a brain-damaged ex-cop/ex-congregant went off his meds and pointed his service weapon at me in anger because I wouldn't "make" his wife come back to him.

This moment in the hallway is scarier than any of that. As if some dark, unknown threat is bearing down on me, unstoppable and malevolent. I beat it to the bathroom and sit under the pedestal sink with the lights off and the door locked. By the time Christie finds me, my heart rate and breathing have slowed, and the sensation passes. A panic attack? When I return to the party, no one is the wiser.

Despite the last year and my diagnosis, I get the feeling no one really understands that these may be our last times together. The last holiday meal, our last drink, our last time to pull out guitars and make music. The holidays highlight this disconnect for me.

On Thanksgiving morning, we're rushing out of the condo to make it to my parent's house on time. I grab a laundry basket with two crockpots of freshly made potatoes – both mashed and sweet - miss a step on the landing and take a head-first tumble down a half-flight of stairs, ending with a header into the front door of the building. The laundry basket hits the floor first and the crock pots launch mushy potatoes – both mashed and sweet – into the air. Christie thinks I've finally succumbed to Sudden Cardiac Death and runs to the stairs to find me sprawled at the bottom in a daze, the walls and my hair festooned with holiday potatoes – both mashed and sweet.

Nothing is broken, but I have some wicked bruising and a persistent headache from the crash. I should have gone to the ER, but since nothing felt broken and it was my last Thanksgiving with family, maybe ever, we go on to my parent's house, late as we are.

Thanksgiving has many times been a buffet style affair with both of our families, but when we arrive to find that everyone has already eaten, we realize again that our loved ones either don't understand or (understandably) didn't want to think about this possibly being one of those "last times." At Christie's house, the same situation, in which conversation and catching up with one another surrenders to the damnable football (Basketball? Tennis? Tetherball?) game. It's not that they don't care. They just aren't processing. I don't blame them. We're not doing a great job of that ourselves. Christmas is a little better, but not much.

Which brings me back to my aversion. I don't let 'em see me sweat, but I have a morbid fear of being the center of attention in a small group. This time, in these moments, I'd hoped for…what? Not necessarily to be fawned over, but for everyone around us to appreciate the gravity of these moments in the same way that we did. In retrospect, we'd already been gone for a year, really for four years before that, living hours away in the Ozarks. Everyone's life has moved on, and we aren't a large part of that anymore. For myself, I feel more like a curiosity than anything else. A window into the world of heart transplants, to be queried and marveled over, then set aside for the next topic of discussion. Maybe that means I want to be the center of attention. I don't know. I only know that while we're glad to have spent time with our family and friends, none of them seem to completely get the fact we might never see one another again. My brother, Darrell, the least likely of people, expresses it to me in a very emotional way the night before we leave. I think my father understands very well, but he's a private person, and like most of us, has trouble expressing big emotions. I'm sure Christie can mention exceptions as well. I just know we drive away certain that even if I make it through this whole thing, we'd rather not settle back in Arkansas. Too much time has passed, and we can't imagine building a life there again, or trying to restore the one we had. The homelessness really starts to sink in. People without a country. Metallica says it best:

> *"...and the earth becomes my throne,*
> *I adapt to the unknown*
> *Under wandering stars I've grown,*
> *by myself but not alone - I ask no one*
> *...and my ties are severed clean,*
> *the less I have the more I gain*
> *Off the beaten path I reign, rover, wanderer*
> *Nomad, vagabond, call me what you will..."*
>
> *(Wherever I May Roam - Metallica)*

A few days after Christmas, the boys with unopened presents and unbuilt Lego sets, we leave for Lebanon, New

Hampshire for a contract at Dartmouth Medical Center. For my part, I doubt I'll see these people, or Arkansas again.

It's hard to imagine building a life anywhere now. We're officially gypsies, on the lam, in every sense of the phrase. In Chris Cornell's final performance on Soundgarden's "King Animal" album, he sings:

"You can't go home, no I swear you never can...
You can walk a million miles and get nowhere.
Got nowhere to go since I've been back...
Just filling in the lines and the holes in the cracks."

(I've Been Away for Too Long - Soundgarden)

He was dead on, and then he was dead. Maybe he thought there was no place for him here anymore. I know the feeling.

Chapter 5

Livestock & Breakables

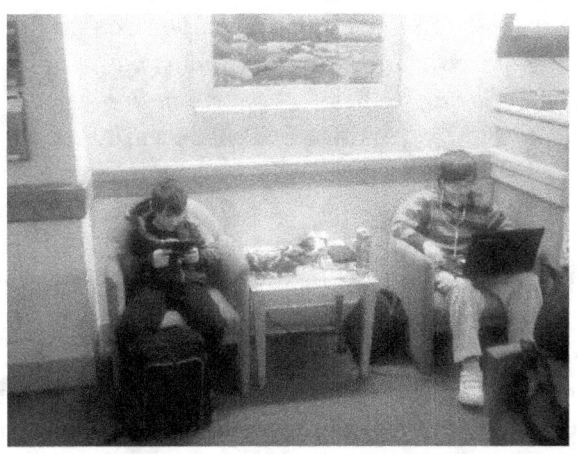

Did you drop it on the floor?
And they told you where it came from there's no more?
Did the pieces cut you when you
tried to sweep them off the ground?
And they told you what is lost cannot be found...
The shelves in here wind like forgotten streets,
and I was born with two left feet,
Porcelain and crystal, everything we bought...
I'm a bull in a china shop

I learned the lesson well when I was young,
Sometimes you just can't finish everything that you've begun,
And confidence sometimes is not enough,
and sometimes life just calls your bluff,
All the glass figurines are spitting lead,

and I'm stumbling around just like the living dead,
The chosen think they're special, even though they're not,
they're all bulls in a china shop

And on and on, the rain will fall, like tears from star,
On and on, the rain will say, how fragile we are,

The bill is due, but my credit's wrecked in here,
where the flesh and spirit melt to liquid fear,
And ending well is all that you can do,
before the burning down consumes you,
All the lies and bluster in the room are cracking,
and our terror's like a hammer with no nail,
The shards are crunching underfoot,
and I can't seem to stop... I'm a bull in a china shop

It's 3:30 am and Rich shifts and pulls one leg up underneath him. He's just tall enough now to cross his arms on the back of the folding chair so he can lay his head on them. Brennan never seemed to master the skill of lap-sitting, so every few minutes, Christie stirs to hoist him back up into her lap, but it'll only take him a few minutes to slide back down again. I can't sleep at all because of the bells and alarms, but mostly because of the A-fib. I'm annoyed that the ER has no more folding chairs, or even an armchair for the boys to sleep in. They've been up since 6 the morning before, when we left the Folsons house in Lebanon, PA.

"*I break everything,*" I think. "*Everybody.*"

The boys should be having friends for sleepovers, not sleeping over in an ER folding chair. I think I've developed a psychosis of sorts. I'm obsessively aware of the myriad ways in which my family has to constantly accommodate, fuss, and suffer for and over me. Is the parking lot too far from the front door? Christie will drop me off and walk back from a quarter of a mile away. In the rain, sometimes. Is it too hot? Is it too heavy to lift? All three of them will do it together while I watch. I'm exhausted and embarrassed. My disease is invisible, and deadly. It's bizarre to those who don't know, and explaining it feels like I'm making excuses for laziness. Psychosis. Another line tumbles through my head... *"I was born with two left feet...stumbling through life like the walking dead..."* I tuck them away in some closet I have in the back of my brain for lyrics. It takes three years before I actually finish the all the words and pull out a guitar.

After saying our goodbyes in Arkansas, we passed through Raleigh, N.C. to visit Mindi (our HCM friend from years ago) and her husband Hugh, one of the honest-to-God best human beings I've ever had the privilege to know. We got to spend some time with our nieces and nephews who lived nearby. From there, we reconnected with the Folsons and made our way on to the perfect New Year's Day in Lebanon, New Hampshire. The quintessential small New England town if there ever was one. The home of Dartmouth Medical Center, Christie's new contract.

We found the apartment, newly built, with furniture already delivered - a relief after the Washingtonvilletownburo debacle. The boys were excited that we had to ride an elevator to the third floor of the sparsely populated building to unload the van. We promised them lots of snow during the New Hampshire winter to come, and New Hampshire didn't disappoint that night. The perfect light snow drifted down through the crisp night air as we entered a small Italian place for a hard-earned dinner. We'd be close enough to Tufts, under two hours, that I could finally be officially listed there. It was the beginning of a new year, a new venture, a new test. Maybe it would also be our new home.

The A-fib arrived just as the food did. I saw my own horror reflected in Christie's face as the blood drained from mine. My stomach turned as the bile began to rise. A searing pain tore through my chest, but I was too weak to clutch at it.

"A-fib," I gasped, as the confused waitress looked on. Christie quickly explained our situation as several other diners turned to see what the gasping was all about. Brennan boxed the food as Christie and Rich got me to my unsteady feet and steered me to the door. It was all I could do not to sink to my knees. I leaned hard on them both as they half-walked, half-dragged me to the van while curious onlookers made a path. I gripped the backs of their chairs and tried to help prop myself using their tables.

Accommodation and fuss.

The broken seesaw sensation in my chest abated for a few moments when we reached the car. I hoped the rhythm had corrected itself - I'm a drummer for crying out loud. But I've also been in the ring with HCM for a long time by now. It never just corrects itself or gets better. It always picks up the sharpest object in the room and aims for your left ventricle. We needed to get to the store to buy toiletries and food, we needed to unpack. The boys, be they ever so patient, are still waiting to open Christmas presents from a week earlier.

"I think it's stopped," I ventured. "Let's go on and see if it comes back."

At the store, I tried to use one of those handicapped carts for the first time. Ever tried to use one of those? They're terrible. I couldn't steer, and every time I backed up, an obnoxiously loud alarm screamed, "HEY! EVERYONE WITHIN EARSHOT! THE HEALTHY LOOKING YOUNG GUY WITH THE SO-CALLED "HEART DISEASE" IS BACKING UP!! LOOK! LOOK!" I swear it did.

When we arrived back at the apartment, I rested for a few seconds with one foot on the ground and one in the van, eyes closed focusing on my heart rhythm. Even my excitement over our new year, our new residence, and possibly our new home couldn't cover it up; I was in full blown Atrial fibrillation.

"Shit!" I yelled. We rarely if ever curse in front of the kids, but I knew what this meant. I'd eaten an appetizer a little over an hour ago. To be cardioverted back into sinus rhythm, I have to be NPO (no food or drink) for at least eight hours. We were going to spend the first night in New Hampshire, after being in limbo for a week and on the road for ten hours, not in our new apartment, but in the ER. We found Dartmouth about five minutes from our parking lot, but this quaint, winter-wonderland town took on a foreboding and sinister edge as Christie wheeled me into the ER for my inevitable sentence. The snow was still gently coming down, but I lost sight of it in the harsh fluorescent lights that washed over us at the entrance.

***

So here I lay, watching my family sleep in folding chairs. I'll tell you so many more painful and difficult things as this story continues, but even on the other side of it all, I still consider this the lowest moment of my entire life. I never did find a way to articulate the way I felt that night, but a friend named Perry (who you'll meet in a future chapter) eventually filled in that blank.

"Everyone around you just wants to have a normal life," he says, "and you just keep tearing everything up. Nothing we can do about it. It's not our fault, but we still do it. It's like that saying...what is it? Bull in a china shop? Of course it's going to break everything! Why is it even there? Who the hell lets a bull into a china shop? It's not the bull's fault, but everything still gets broken."

Livestock and breakables. Never a good mix. Life is fragile and has very little room for people who go careening around like a kid in a bouncy house. Someone eventually gets hurt, and it's usually not the kid who's flailing around with his shoes still on.

After six hours of insistence that the ER docs call Boston, they finally do. I'm cardioverted and stabilized, but the docs won't let me go. They admit me to a shared room in a loud and busy hallway where I try to sleep after having been awake for twenty-six hours at that point. Christie and the boys go back to sleep at the apartment and deal with the details. In the morning, I argue again with the cardiology team, then Christie arrives and wins a shout-down with the know-it-all attending cardiologist over my fluid retention.

"This isn't fat," he yells at her, jiggling my bloated belly. "It's water, and it needs to come off."

She raises her voice to meet his volume. "We KNOW THAT! He's hypertrophic! We just moved here from Arkansas yesterday because of it! He's being seen by the HCM guys at Tufts in two weeks! We don't NEED your help!"

He throws his hands up, but I threaten to leave AMA (against medical advice). If he tries to get this fluid off of my abdomen, he'll kill me. Rapid duiresing of an HCM patient can literally cause the entire vascular system to cave in on itself. He gives up and finally releases me the next evening. We go home in the dark.

My heart repeats this same set of shenanigans a week later, again at a restaurant, again after I've just eaten and have to wait all night. The only difference is that the boys have at least been able to open the rest of their presents, and the ER nurse was kind enough to bring in two reclining chairs for the family to sleep in. I still haven't seen anything of Lebanon, New Hampshire during the day except the apartment parking lot. I worry that too much exertion will bring on the A-fib again, but it doesn't matter. It happens a third time, but instead of rushing to the ER, I wait out my time at home, while everyone gets some sleep, binge watching episodes of David Simon's new show "Treme" on some pirated website. When it's time, we leave the boys connected to the Folson's via Skype and run up the street for another run-of-the-mill cardioversion. It's the first time we've ever left them home by themselves, and it's worrisome, but our friends stay connected with them and we're home in a few hours, my chest feeling like it's been French-fried.

It's almost a month before I actually feel well enough to get out and see the town. It reminds me of Aviano, the small town in northern Italy where my dad was assigned in the early 80's. Surrounded by snow-covered mountains, cool, but not bitter weather. There's a robust home-school network though we never really manage to make any friends – we're here temporarily after all – and there's more to do with the boys than we have time for. They fall in love with the nearby indoor pool park, as well as the modest but impressive science museum on the edge of town. The restaurants are fantastic and diverse, especially considering how small the town is. We discover Argentinian and Nepalese cuisine and become regulars at an Irish pub near the apartment. I talk the boys into learning to play Dungeons & Dragons, an unfulfilled passion of mine since junior high school (yes, I was one of the cool kids). It passes the time while Christie works, and during her days off, we travel to Vermont, visit the cider mills, and the glass shops. New Hampshire doesn't live up to the winter hype that year though – it's the driest season on recent record and most of the ski slopes and sledding trails are closed due to lack of snow cover. There's so many other things to do that it doesn't matter.

I'm blogging in earnest now and trying to chronicle our travels so the boys can have a record of it all when they're older. I name the blog "News of My Demise," from the famous Mark Twain line, "the news of my death has been greatly exaggerated." I try to focus on what's happening with us, our explorations and my health, delving into the world of HCM, transplants, the medical and financial struggles that accompany it all, and my thoughts on chronic illness. The boys both got laptops during our time in Little Rock, which they desperately needed for our homeschooling, and spend a lot of time playing games and tinkering around and experimenting with different programs.

When the time comes to go to Boston, we face a new dilemma; we don't have anyone to leave the boys with if I have to stay overnight in the hospital. The obvious solution is for Christie to just spend the night with them in the hotel across the street from

Tufts, but we're both extremely worried about me being in a hospital without her there. If not for her intervention on several occasions in Arkansas ER's, I'd have been dead years ago. We'd like to hope that Tufts is different, but we don't know. Just because Dr. Maron and the HCM clinic are there doesn't necessarily mean the ER or the Electrophysiology labs are HCM savvy. The Folsons agree to meet us in Boston and take the boys should my electrical study require an overnight admission, but they have to cancel the night before due to a meeting at work. We head for Boston the next morning with no idea how the situation is going to play out. Christie is terrified of leaving me alone overnight, but the boys can't stay by themselves either. We're reminded again of just how alone we are all the way up here, out of reach of family and friends.

Our worrying is in vain - the renowned HCM electrophysiologist, Dr. Link, puts me on a regimen of anti-arrhythmic medications and there's no need to stay overnight for the workup.

"The Amiodarone should hold you for a while," he says, "but the A-fib will come back. It always comes back."

"Then what?" I ask.

"Then we have to start burning out cellular nodes with a laser to kill the malfunctioning sections of wiring. That's only going to work for so long in your case. You need a new heart."

By the middle of February, we've made three or four trips to Tufts and I've completed tests to be listed for transplant. We spend the rest of the assignment exploring nearby Maine and fall in love with Portsmouth, a small town full of artisans and crab shacks along the coast. We eat our way from there all the way down to the northside of Boston one weekend, our road winding along the Atlantic coastline. We spend a lot of time in Boston, mixing business with pleasure. Doctor appointments with Dr. Maron and Dr. Kiernan, the transplant guy, then off to the Boston

Aquarium or Paul Revere's house in Little Italy. I'm doing my best to join our history lessons with what we're seeing there.

I think we could live here in Lebanon, New Hampshire. In the quiet solitude of the infrequent snowfalls, the small towns with pre-colonial churches and universities, and the looming mountains all around, promising some new sight.

The vistas here are truly breathtaking at times and as much as we need to be close to our families and friends during all this, the beauty and newness of it all nearly makes up for the struggles of being alone. We're beginning to have more confidence in ourselves, that we can handle whatever curve balls are thrown at us.

Our next assignment challenges that notion yet again.

***

By the time Dartmouth offers Christie a full-time position, we're committed to Norwalk, Connecticut, and off we go.

It is the worst of all possible assignments. Though the HCM is quiet and I get news that I am finally listed at Tufts, Christie works eight-hour swing shifts, effectively trapping me and the boys at our small apartment most days. When she's off, the traffic is so terrible that it takes all day to navigate the grocery store, the post office, and library. It's so chaotic that our nightly dinner ritual is abandoned, and we barely see each other. Attempts to find homeschool co-ops are fruitless in that city made up of young professionals commuting to Manhattan every day of the week, and everything closes at eight because the crime rate is so high. Christie fights depression because of the negligence and recklessness at the hospital and is continually in conflict with doctors and administration who expect her to look the other way. Despite a few retreats to New York City and visits with the Folsons, we feel isolated, disconnected, and listless. I'm finally listed, but what now? We've worked toward this one thing for the last two years and now whatever happens is out of our hands. I spend most of my days working through math courses on Kahn Academy, partly because I've taken over paying the bills and partly because the thought of creative pursuits depresses me. I try to take up painting but lose interest. I write a single song (Thru the Storm) that ends up on my Instead of Wither album. Otherwise, I'm dry. We all are.

We can't get out of there fast enough, despite the offer of a full-time job. Baystate Medical Center in Springfield, Massachusetts has a contract in thoracic IMC that may turn into a full-time position. It's under two hours from Boston, so we sign on, sight unseen. We're not excited about the location, but it meets our needs for a transplant situation and it feels like maybe our years on the road are coming to an end.

All the stories about people lost in the desert seeing a fresh oasis only realize it's merely a mirage? I hate those stories.

Chapter 6

Twist

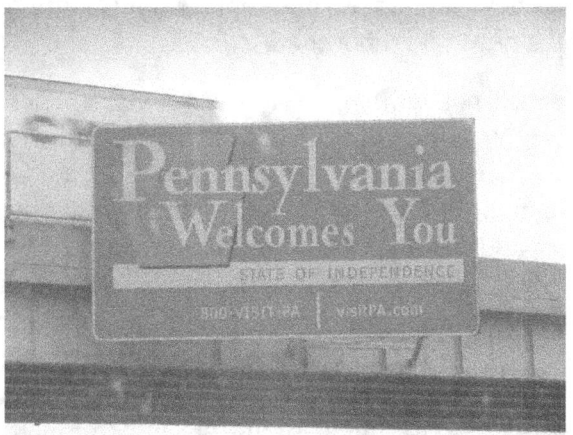

Freewill, wasted on the bound, I can't get my head around,
Double speak, displace the meek, find shelter, find Summerland,
I will not beg your pardon, I will not bribe or barter,
Pack my bags and leave

Come a time to stand your ground and bleed,
Come a time to cut your losses,
In the end nothing to defend,
Leave a man, twisting in the wind

Lowdown promises to break, not much more that I can take,
On the sly, a dirty lie, don't cower, but don't bite the hand,
I will not stand on virtue, I never meant to hurt you,
Pack my bags and leave,

"It's a cool place to live, but people sometimes complain about the noise," the kid tells us. He can't be twenty yet, but he's showing us the apartment Christie's company has rented for us in Springfield, Massachusetts. He blows the hair out of his eyes and tries to turn on the kitchen lights. "Must need a bulb," he mumbles.

And a coat of paint, I think, looking around the dilapidated kitchen. And new appliances, and replacement flooring. And new carpet. And a new...neighborhood.

"Yeah, I noticed the bar across the street. Lots of bikes," Christie says. We're comfortable with bikers and spent a lot of time around them while in ministry with Calvary Chapel. But bikers come in all flavors and we know Banditos and Angels from Rock Riders and Saviors. These aren't the kind of bikers we're used to. We passed a hopper (corner boy – low man on the drug business totem) in the apartment courtyard on the way in. This isn't necessarily a worry for Christie and me, drugs and trafficking being familiar territory from our time in ministry. But drugs mean guns, and guns mean bullets flying around, through windows, walls, cars...children...

I pull Brennan a little closer and note the broken blinds in most of the windows. Dead flies fill the windowsills. The heat is stifling.

"They have to call the cops out most nights on the weekends. Fights and stuff. There's a new curfew but nobody keeps to it." He seems amused and even a little proud of this.

I know these places. I've been here many times. The beleaguered owner, standing behind a hotel style desk, watching who comes and goes. Keeping track of the people on their way into or out of rehab. He might be questioned by the cops about them at some point. The local AA and NA will be a constant presence, and I spot the flyers on the way out of the lobby. People working temp jobs and odd shifts. Noisy, dirty, unpredictable.

Christie's company has had a difficult time taking care of us in the housing department from the beginning. Danville, furniture problems in New Hampshire, bad location in Connecticut. Now this. Travel nurses usually go it alone, single people seeing the country, with little other concern. For a family of four, one of which can't climb stairs to the second or third floor, it's tougher to find three-month leases. The situation has been precarious, but this is over the edge.

Luckily, I'd looked at some pictures on Google Earth (since the complex didn't even have a web site) and got a feel for the address. Bad vibes. We've taken the Saturday prior to re-assignment to drive up from Norwalk to check it out. Good thing. I spend the rest of the week working with the company's housing department to find something else. But there isn't much. I learn later that the residents of Springfield have a saying; "Springfield. Come for the Night Life, Stay Because You Got Murdered."

I end up finding a remodeled apartment that used to serve as a Remington factory in the downtown area. It's part of an effort to clean up the city's worsening drug problem, and it seems safe. They don't contract with Christie's company, so we negotiate our own deposit and they work out the rest with the company. The apartment complex is clean, but I'm all too familiar with these parts of towns from my days of ministry in Little Rock and club gigs with various bands. We barely get furniture leased and delivered in time and make the moving deadline with only a few minutes to spare.

The next three months blur by. Christie's parents visit, we continue to homeschool, but we're all exhausted and ready to get off the road. When the hospital offers Christie a job, we take it and immediately start looking for rent houses and exploring the possibility of buying a home. In the end we find a rental in a suburb, and by October we're settled in. When we'd been in Little

Rock over the holidays, my family helped us get our belongings out of the emergency storage (remember the snowstorm the day we left Bentonville?) and get to my in-law's garage. Now, Christie's family loads it onto a trailer and her folks drive it north to us. A local band contacts me from some ancient Google profile and I audition to sing, but with the understanding that my ability to perform live and travel is extremely limited. They're more interested in recording a demo, so I sign on. Maybe we'll find some semblance of normal life here for a while, now that we're where we need to be.

But all I feel is numb. Depression? Acceptance? For me, Springfield is a vast plain of monochromatic nothingness punctuated by brief bursts of creativity. It should feel good to have some stability, a predictable schedule, and some normalcy. I'm surrounded by familiar things, haven't had A-fib in over a year, and I'm able to be transplanted, blood type and HCM notwithstanding. We've done all we can do. But I'm cold and empty, lost in this strange place with no friends or connections. Where is Springfield? Who am I here? Who are we?

It feels like a waiting room to me, the backstage green room where there's nothing more to do but keep re-tuning guitars and nit-picking the breaches in the contract rider. We're only here for me to get a transplant. Try as I might, we can't find any significant homeschooling presence in the area; of course, Massachusetts is known for having the most well-funded and successful education system in the nation, so why homeschool? The boys prefer it anyway but I'm unmotivated, relying mostly on workbooks and online instruction. I don't push much when they procrastinate or shy away from projects. It's my fault we're here, in this social wasteland, with no friends or connections. I feel guilty disciplining them or forcing them to do anything they don't want to. They've had their fair share of that. I shouldn't be disconnected like this, but I can't stir up enough vision or passion to invest in much of anything.

The band is an on-again-off-again prospect, revolving members and such. I get to write and sing some original material for an EP, which gets some creative juices flowing. When I have the notion, I work on a novel I've been pecking away at for the last five years about the Medici family. I take some online cooking classes. Christie works second job two days a week and seems happy. I expected to feel some sense of accomplishment or…something, now that we've achieved our goal of getting within view of Boston. But it's not the city we'd have chosen to live in, not by a long-shot. I've lost any vision of what "home" looks like to me anymore, or what I'm doing with myself. HCM has pushed me around for so long, I almost don't know what to do without it dictating to me.

Maybe I'm just tired. More than anything, I wonder how I came to be in this foreign place, devoid of personality, art, a music scene, or friendships. I'm worn out, physically, emotionally, psychologically. Following his divorce, my good friend Smitty once asked me, "do you ever look around and wonder 'how is this my life?' Not in a bad way, but just wondering how everything became so unfamiliar. The people and places you thought would always be there are gone or changed, and you feel like a stranger in your own life." Yeah. I do that every day now.

In November of 2012 I start to have sinus infections and a sore throat that won't go away. It interferes with my singing voice and live performances with the band all the way into the following February. I play some video games, but spend most of my time watching throw-away television – Curtis Stone's Take Home Chef, and Queer Eye for the Straight Guy. The latter leaves me fascinated with the notion that life is right enough for some guys that they think about things like their hair and the way they dress. Maybe I used to care about those things to some degree, when I was going to be on stage. I know who I am as a husband and father, but my personal identity has been stripped down to nothing. I wear no jewelry, my wedding ring the only real personal effect. I'm in pajama pants and slippers most days. Why not? I have nowhere to go, no one to see. I don't even connect with, Blitzy, the sweet little dog we adopt after moving in. She reminds me of the beginning of this whole train wreck, back in 2010, finding Nanouq that morning in a puddle of her own urine. There's a metaphor there but I can't pinpoint it. The boys become fixated on Minecraft and I give up schooling them all together in the early spring semester. I can't blame them for not wanting to spend time doing school – they're kids. Even more, it means they have to spend time with me. And I don't even want to do that.

My fluid retention gets noticeably worse over the holidays, and not because I'm eating too much. I don't have an appetite anymore, even with the time I'm spending learning to cook and experimenting with gourmet recipes. My calls and emails to Boston are starting to go unanswered. The coordinator that we loved and trusted has passed us off to her assistant who doesn't know our journey thus far. Dr. Maron, who I trust with my life, has been forced to pass me to the transplant team, and Dr. Michael Kiernan. Neither Christie or I trust him because he tries to avoid saying the hard things and doesn't look me in the eye when his hand is forced. In turn, he's passed me off to his Fellow, and we're fighting the same battle we did in Arkansas.

"You're probably gaining because of sodium. Cut down on your salt intake."

"You're getting older, it's not uncommon to gain weight."

"Your echo looks the same as it did last year. Your symptoms shouldn't be worse."

I'm too exhausted to argue, but I know that I'm progressing again. Good. Maybe I'll move up the list and we can get this over with. Or maybe I won't, and it will at least be over for my family, and they can get on with their lives. I'm sick of it all, sick of myself, sick of being sick with no end in sight.

***

Valentine's Day, 2013. Although I drive into Boston for infrequent appointments on my own, we all go that day, drawn by the growing popularity of an oyster and lobster roll bar near the hospital. Christie and I arrive determined to have it out with Kiernan about being passed off to a Fellow who seems HCM ignorant and discuss the increased fluid retention. Turns out there's no need.

Kiernan comes in, fidgety and distracted. Flustered. He's a young guy, very tall, with a well-meaning but somewhat awkward bedside manner.

"So, your echo is a bit worse. I think you're at the point where we can just call this heart failure now. I don't know that the HCM part is relevant to the bigger picture moving forward because the burn-out brings you under the larger umbrella of general heart failure. It's significant and progressive."

I wish someone would write a new verse for this same old tired song.

"The problem is, I'm not sure what to do for you. We have a really bad situation on our cardiac ICU. There are a dozen people who've been living here for over a year, waiting, and most of them are O-Positive. There's just not enough organs being donated, even less than usual. I think it's fortunate with your work situation that you can travel to other places, because that's the best advice I can give you - move. There are a few centers that would meet your needs, one in North Carolina, another near Los Angeles. Would you be able to get to one of those?"

What's the point of explaining to him that we've spent two and a half years struggling to get within driving distance of the room we're sitting in right now? That Christie had just five months earlier signed a year-long job contract? That we'd signed a twelve-month rental lease? That we'd gotten a dog and weren't travelling anymore? That the kids had their own rooms and a routine? That I'd joined a band (sort of)? That Christie's parents had driven a trailer all the way from Arkansas to bring our belongings to us? I was tired of explaining anything anymore. How would he even begin to grasp the magnitude of what he was telling us? For starters, we'd had to pay a $1400 deposit for the home we were renting. Probably a drop in the bucket for a heart transplant specialist in his mid-20's living in Boston. Why bother trying to explain it? It wouldn't have changed my listing status by a micrometer. It wouldn't change anything. Chronic illness leaves you no one to complain to. Some people blame God, or their version of God, but you may as well blame the sky or the sea. It changes nothing.

We went to the rather forgettable oyster bar and ate okay-ish lobster rolls (but they get a pass - I was distracted). Another $60 for a Boston lunch. I ate mostly salad because I couldn't afford the salt, but more so because I was sick to my stomach. We'd been turned away from how many transplant programs now? But this was Tufts. This was Dr. Marty Maron and the HCM clinic. The Mecca of HCM treatment on the planet. We should be safe here. This is the solution, the goal. So why are we standing outside the walls staring up at the locked gate?

***

It's not Marty's fault, obviously. No one can fight UNOS, or the organ shortage. It feels like betrayal, and here we are again, just like St. Louis, with nothing to show for our efforts except wasted time and increasing credit card debt. Downtown Boston isn't cheap, and we've spent nearly two years now in overpriced hotels, overpriced restaurants, and buying Charlie passes (for the subway). A hotel within any reasonable distance of the hospital is $230 per night, easily. For another $40 we can stay right across the street from the hospital and save the $50 on cabs that day. Meals for four people average about $100, and that's nowhere fancy. But it's tough for someone avoiding sodium like the plague to eat fast food all the time, and all the activity means I needed massive amounts of protein for fuel, so salads only go so far. A non-eventful visit to Tufts with tests one day and appointments the next, runs us anywhere from $600 - $800 by the time we get in and out, more than that if Christie misses work to come, since we will be short that income. We make sandwiches as much as we can, especially for day trips now that we live close enough. At an average of one visit every three weeks, we've watched our credit card debt climb to around $25,000 without a cent going to actual medical bills. A chunk of that is left over from our fruitless trips to St. Louis in 2010.

I guess we could be blamed for trying to do something fun or educational with the kids when we make these trips, over and over, from 2010 to 2013. We aren't extravagant. A water park here, a museum there. A candy store if we pass one. Part of our trying to balance things out. They spend so much time sitting quietly and reading or playing on their laptops in waiting rooms and hospital cafeterias. Hours, multiple days sometimes, until they know the staff on a first name basis and look forward to seeing them. For Christie and I, doing something fun with them afterwards goes a long way towards taking the edge off the anxiety, restoring some joy, and providing brief shelters of distraction from the torrent of dread that pours continually. A bit of added debt is a small price to pay for that relief, and it seems to remind the kids that there is more to life than my illness, despite how much it has dictated our lives. And here we are, being dictated to again.

This never sits well with Christie, to whom no one, including HCM, is the boss of. Her ability to rebound, adjust, and move forward is rivaled only by my psychological and emotional confusion in these moments. By the time we've driven the hour and a half home, she has a plan to grab the UNOS database by the throat and squeeze until it gives up some piece of crucial information that will point to our next step.

It amazes me still as I speak with so many transplant candidates that they are largely unaware of how organ procurement and the so called "waiting list" actually work. They are content to simply wait in ignorant bliss until the call comes - and remain so even after the surgery. But we can't wait. We know that many people with HCM and the added misfortune of an O positive blood type, die waiting. Ignorant bliss isn't my style either; I find immense comfort in data, numbers, and understanding of how something like the UNOS database works. It fascinates me on some sociological level. Most people imagine a long waiting list where names are checked off the top as organs become available, and everyone else moves up a spot. I regret that it isn't that simple, and so will you by the time I finish explaining it. Feel free to catch a quick nap in the middle.

In reality, the country is divided into several zones or "regions," and there is a given number of transplant centers in each zone for various organs. Each zone has its own list, which fluctuates due to many factors; transplants, deaths while waiting, changing urgency, changing time accumulated, and removal because of ineligibility, usually due to sickness or non-compliance. The list is in constant flux, shaped by the forces that play themselves out in the lives of thousands who wait. When things started to get real, we learned how to use the filter systems on the database and educated ourselves on what the numbers meant. We learned how to get hard numbers on how many people were listed in a given zone, which hospitals had high and low populations of transplant candidates, the primary, secondary, and tertiary conditions for which they are listed, their genders, blood types - and even optional phenotype classes - and time accumulated on the list. We could also interpret the data to understand survival rates, rate of transplants, and how many had been transplanted in a given time frame, for what, how long they'd waited, average survival rates following transplant, re-transplantation...bored yet?

So, we throw down with the UNOS database as soon as we get home that night. The hospitals Dr. Kiernan had suggested are a no-go. They've transplanted some HCM patients, but not many, and their wait times aren't stellar. We start cross-referencing, filtering, trimming the fat, trying to tease this one bit of information out of the unwieldy monster. Then finally, we're down to two places, one in California. The other is like a familiar face, smiling up at us from the screen.

Hershey, Pennsylvania.

***

Hershey, Pennsylvania? Didn't we just leave that party?

First, we call our friends, the Folsons, to discuss the possibility of staying with them while we look for rentals in the area. We're excited at the possibility of moving back – we loved the people and slower pace of life, the dairy farms, and homeschool co-op were we still stayed in touch with many friends. We don't say anything to the boys or anyone else until we know it will work for sure. No one needs another disappointment, least of all the boys.

The next day, I start digging. First up, Lisa Salberg at the HCMA.

"Who's treating patients at Penn State?" I ask.

"Oh, that's Eric. He comes to our conventions, he's spoken several times. Eric Popjes."

Yep, it's pronounced just like it looks. I still use his name gratuitously just so I can pop the "P" at the front. Sometimes there's spittle.

I explain the situation to her, and she's not wild about the idea of a transplant at Hershey. The survival rate is marginal. We want it to work so badly, but depending on the circumstances of the deaths, it can be a deal-breaker. The thought of moving all the way to the heat of North Carolina or the far-distant land of California is almost unbearable.

Lisa connects me to Aaron, a twenty-something year old post-transplant patient from Hershey. Though I've long forgotten his last name, I'll be forever grateful to him. He was only a few weeks out from the surgery but sounded fantastic.

"Popjes is the man! He's been taking care of me since I was a kid," Aaron tells me. "Got diagnosed with HCM when I was eight. He kept me alive all this time, got me transplanted. I owe the guy my life a couple of times over."

"What about these deaths? From the math, it looks like they've had three right in a row recently."

"A mom and daughter. I knew them," he says. "They were transplanted right around the same time, both went into rejection about the same time. You never know with things like that. Could have been something they ate. Maybe they weren't compliant. You gotta be compliant if you want to live."

Compliance is a big deal in the transplant world, before and after. Not complying with fluid and diet restrictions can cause Bad Things to happen that might put you in a suspended status on the list (the dreaded "Status Seven"). If your kidney function falters too much, or your liver fails, you're not a good candidate. Afterward, your immune system is suppressed to the point that the common cold can kill you if left unattended. Taking meds on time, staying hydrated, being compliant. Your life is absolutely dependent on it.

I learn later that the reason Hershey has such a bad survival rate is because they tend to take high-risk patients that probably shouldn't have been listed in the first place. This turns out to be a good thing for me.

We make a cardiology appointment as soon as they can get me in. Then we tell the boys what's happening. We expect a tumult of cheers and a lot of jumping around. We've been spending any significant vacation time back in Lebanon and Annville, Pennsylvania, visiting friends and staying with the Folsons. Playing with the Folson kids is their favorite thing, and they're online with them every waking second that they're not doing chores.

Brennan slowly begins to cry. Rich doesn't say anything, just stares at us, his expression blank. They've been isolated here, with no friends, no amenities – there is no swimming pool, skating rink, park, homeschool group…nothing. Of all the places they'd want to live, it would be near Hershey.

Brennan's quiet weeping escalates into wailing. We're consoling him and utterly confused. Rich calmly says, "That would be awesome. I'm just tired of moving."

"What about you?" Christie asks Brennan.

"I don't want to move," he sobs. Gut-wrenching, shoulder shaking sobs. I can't remember ever seeing him so upset.

"Why not?" we all must have asked in unison. He matches our confusion with exasperation.

"Number one," he began, counting on his fingers, "we JUST moved here. Number two, I like our house. Number three, Blitzy likes this house. Number four, mom has to change jobs. Number five, we JUST got all of our stuff here and unpacked. Number FIVE, what about fencing? Number SIX, what about Rich's archery?" He continued, raising his voice. "Number SIX, we're going to be even FARTHER away from Arkansas. Number NINE, we just learned where everything is here, Number twelve…" He finally runs out of steam and starts sobbing again.

First of all, I lose a few points here for geography education (and maybe math…) because in his mind, Pennsylvania was farther away from Arkansas than Massachusetts. But I think I should get a pass on the number skipping. He was upset.

Secondly, like someone punching me in the stomach, I realize that in Brennan's mind, he's holding on to some notion that we'll eventually return to Arkansas, that we're somehow obligated to it, and that the farther away from it we travel, the harder it will be to ever get back to the life that had been so stable and predictable to him. I realize I'm holding on to the same fantasy. Nothing from Bentonville has been replaced. The places he and I used to spend our time, the library, the gym, the park, are gone, and Springfield offers no semblance of replacement for them. We both want to go back, for things to just go back to the way they were. This move will be yet another step away from that fantasy.

He's comforted by the reminder that we all have friends there, that we won't be so alone, like we are here. We remind him of Hershey Park, Cleona park, the library, Patches creamery and the farmer's markets. He doesn't realize we can take Blitzy with us, that Christie can go back to the job she had before. We manage to calm and reassure him, but I know that his distress isn't about any of those specific things. He's just exhausted from the never-ending uprooting and travel. He carries the weight of my heart failure on him more heavily than I want to believe. But in moments like these, I can see the burden clearly.

I spent a lot of time hiding in the bathroom that day. Bull in a china shop again. I hate the saying "kids are resilient." I don't think they are. I think tell ourselves that to assuage the guilt of putting the needs of life, and often our own needs, in front of theirs. That supposed resiliency certainly isn't reflected in our society full of adults with adjustment disorders, anxiety, anger management problems, and fear of the unknown. Even now, writing this nearly four years after this incident, I can see the effects the instability has had on him. He is a staunch creature of habit, not unwilling to try new things, but satisfied to stay within his comfort zone, and wary of big changes. Rich is even more like this in some regards.

The relocation is a nightmare within a nightmare. Lebanon, where we're looking for a rental, is a twelve-hour round trip from Springfield. We make two, three-day trips using Christie's remaining PTO days, looking for a rental, but there are none to be found, at least, none in a safe part of town. We turn to a friend we'd made through the Folsons, Marc Gecker. He's a realtor near the end of his career in his late sixties, but he digs in hard and starts coming up with some places we might be able to buy, given our specific needs. Most houses in our price range in that area are two story, a problem in and of itself since stairs are my nemesis. So we need a downstairs bathroom. More than one climb a day and I'm done. We also need a room, be it dining, office, or living, that can be closed off to use as a bedroom should my condition deteriorate to a bed-ridden state before transplant. Unlikely. The thing Christie and I both know but don't say is that if the transplant takes too long, or I get a heart and have rejection, we need a room for me to die in. One where I can have privacy, not climb stairs, and get myself back and forth to the bathroom on my own for as long as I can. So many things can go wrong, and the reality is, we need something that would work for a hospice situation.

Our initial consult with the head of Cardiology, Dr. Dwight Davis goes extremely well. He's warm, intelligent, and doesn't candy-coat (a prime requisite for us by now). He seems to know more about fluid retention than anyone we've ever met and lays out a plan for getting me into the system, transferring my wait time from Tufts over to HMC (Hershey Medical Center), and makes sure we're all on the same page about the trajectory for my HCM and the transplant process. We don't get to meet Dr. Popjes, but Dr. Davis seems to have everything in hand.

Marc does his best through April and May during our hit-and-run trips to Lebanon, but we're not finding anything that will work. The dual-edged sword is that although Christie has a job waiting on her in Hershey, she has to start orientation on July 5th with a group of new hires, or she has to wait until the next group, sometime in September. We're already hand to mouth trying to come up with loan deposit and deal with moving expenses so quickly after travelling. Two months without a paycheck translates to homelessness at this point. She's being released from her contract in Springfield on the 3rd of July, two days before, on the condition that she completes her week's shifts. Our landlord has also graciously released us from our lease after only nine months, with a promise of our deposit back. But he's already scheduled someone to move in on the 5th of July.

It plays out like this: We have no house or job in Springfield as of the 5th of July. Christie has to start work in Hershey on the 6th of July – and here's the kicker – she must be able to verify a permanent physical address in the state of Pennsylvania. This seems odd to us until she's told that the hospital has issues with employees from out of state and conflicts between labor laws and union policies. A P.O. Box won't do, and we aren't comfortable asking friends to let us use their address. Bottom line, we have to find a house, and we have to have our deposit money from the rental in Springfield to do it. And it has to happen on the 4th or 5th of July. The 4th is a holiday. Meaning our target to move is the 4th, and we must close on the 5th. If we don't close, Christie has no job, not to mention, we're sitting in Lebanon, PA with all of our earthly belongings in the back of a twenty-eight-foot moving van that we're renting by the day, and nowhere to live. We surely could have stayed with the Folsons, or even the Geckers (our realtor Marc, and his wife Ellen with whom we'd become fast friends) for a few days. But what then? To make matters worse, we had to get an FHA loan because of our debt to income ratio, and they're known to be very ticky about closing conditions.

June arrives and a one-off trip to Lebanon lands us in a gorgeous two story in a decent part of town. "The Pershing Place" we still call it, wistfully. It smells of cat, a problem easily remedied as we planned to tear out the carpet and refinish the wood floors before we even unpack (the one handyman skill I actually possess). It has a separate apartment upstairs for visiting parents, a space for homeschooling, and potential room for a small music studio. The kitchen was a dream and the backyard is Blitzy sized, just in need of a reasonable chain link fence to keep her from chasing squirrels into traffic. Our search is over, with plenty of time to spare. We all love the place and head home to Springfield relieved to have found something that meets our needs in the right price range. Marc is confident our bid will be accepted without negotiation, so we make the six-hour drive back to Springfield, our shoulders feeling just a bit less burdened.

Except that the house wasn't actually on the market, Marc calls to inform me later that night. It's in short-sale with the bank and the realtor had it listed wrong. Short-sale sounds like a good thing to me until Marc explains that banks will drag their feet for years before actually selling a house they've repossessed. As of this writing, four years later, "The Pershing Place" is still in short-sale by the bank.

I swear I hear the ominous ticking of a clock. Christie doesn't have any days off for the next two weeks. Even if we find something on our next trip down, it gives us two weeks to close. We start packing and I finish up the EP recording with the band (Mental Pause). We spend three more days in Lebanon looking at every house that has indoor plumbing (well, it isn't that bad, but our criteria had become much more pliable). We just need a roof over our heads at this point. We end up looking at nearly thirty houses over the course of those days, until finally, the last one, late on the third day, feels right. A little New England bungalow on Oak St. A generous front porch with a downstairs bath and isolated dining room, just in case. It's small, too small for us, and we only have 15 minutes to poke around. But it's cozy, close to the hospital and our homeschool friends, and feels more like home than anything we've seen since The Pershing Place (an forever unrequited love story…)

I average four hours of sleep a night for the next two weeks, battling with FHA over the closing arrangements. We agree to pay the asking price and discover that the sellers have a similar deadline approaching in Delaware around the 5th. I'm on the phone with Marc and my poor father daily, begging for advice to navigate the FHA nonsense. The financial officer at the realty company tries to move the closing date several times. FHA wants an expensive chimney repair, a radon system upgrade, and on and on it goes, each repair negotiated between us and the seller, neither having the funds to do much of anything. It all comes together about three days before the planned move. Or so I think.

"The exterior paint on the outside of the house is flaking everywhere," the FHA inspector complains to me on the phone. "It needs to be stripped and repainted."

"In a week? That's impossible!" I'm a wreck from the stress and being up late with Christie trying to work out logistics of moving and paperwork, along with packing, which I'm not able to do much of by now. Plus, summer is here and the temperatures outside are rising, and like most places in Massachusetts, we have no central air conditioning. We'd moved in during October, had a cozy winter, and have now discovered, with much alarm and cursing, that the single window in the living room is in the only one that can accommodate an air conditioner. Good thing we're moving; heat is not my friend. I'm already having trouble breathing in normal temperatures. This new roadblock with the paint nearly sends me over the edge.

I spend two days on the phone begging painters to work over the July 4th weekend - but only one would even consider it, after I offer to pay extra (which we can't afford to do). He looks at the house, concludes that it's lead paint, and needs to be tented, tarped, and stripped in HVAC suits due to the lead content (how he knows this from sight, I have no idea, and I can't contest him - I've not even walked all the way around the outside of the place. I'm in Massachusetts). He's even willing to put the enormous bill on payments, but there's no way he can finish before closing on the 5th.

What now? I plead with FHA. Can we sign something saying we'll do it within a week of move in? Is there any way around this? Of course not.

No recourse - we call Marc and tell him the deal is off. We're Pennsylvania bound, like it or not. With no home to go to, Christie also has no job. At the very least, we have to find a storage unit for our furniture (again) until we figure out what to do. We have to be out by the 5th, and we can't rent a moving van indefinitely. Bleak hardly describes that day. Do we crawl back to Arkansas, tail between legs, and hope family or friends will take us in? Going back to the south is a death sentence for me. I spend the next day trying to find a storage unit and condo or short-term stay that would allow dogs in Lebanon, Pennsylvania. Christie and I refuse to get rid of Blitzy – we've promised the boys a dog once we got settled and there's no way I'm taking it away now, after everything else. Possibly a foolish hill to die on for an adult, but to my mind, this is where I draw the line. I'm sick and tired of watching them lose one thing after another in all of this. I finally find storage, something tiny, away from town, but it isn't large enough to accommodate our belongings.

Then, salvation. The seller's realtor relays that they have to sell the house and are determined to have it painted and ready for closing on the 5th! Christie and I cry with relief, though still worried that FHA with their notorious shenanigans will botch the closing, thus botching Christie's job. I rage at our situation - at our age, the lifestyle we live, we should be able to get a traditional loan and not fool with FHA, but we aren't financially secure enough. Why not? Because I've not worked in fifteen years and we've racked up massive credit card debt making useless trips to St. Louis and Boston. Why? Because of this damn disease ... and I'm suffering the pain of the stress every day, chest tightness and constant angina.

I could write an entire other book chronicling Christie's hardship throughout this journey, even up to this point (and they will become more intense before the end); hating change so much she vomited every morning before leaving for orientation for yet a new contract job. Carrying seven 16x14x14 heavily packed plastic bins, two-weeks clothing for the family, and the kid's 4-

tower Lego collection in and out of apartments, up and down stairs every three months, doing all the grocery shopping after working 12 hour night shifts, working two jobs on numerous occasions, staying up an additional 10 hours to go with me to doctor appointments and tests, the distance from her father who has been battling cancer for over a decade, being separated from her grandmother during the final years of her life…

But at this point, the move from Springfield to Lebanon, Pennsylvania is the most physically demanding of her. She is obligated by contract to work her remaining shifts at Bay State Med Center in Springfield, so no calling off to pack or move. She works three-twelve-hour shifts in a row, then, comes home and begins loading the moving van. We've hired two guys to help load the truck, but she inevitably works harder than them both. We're packed by noon, moving van and the Honda, and on the road to Lebanon, PA. We arrive at the Folson's in time for fireworks and sleep uncomfortably on the futon that night, just grateful for a place to sleep at all. Who knows what tomorrow will bring?

We rise early to meet with Marc for final paperwork and the closing. All goes well, though I hold my breath the entire time. When we arrive at the house, the seller barely acknowledges us as he trots out the front door with a few last belongings in his arms. Curious behavior but it only takes ten minutes to discover why.

No one should ever buy a house sight-unseen. Only looking at it for ten minutes prior isn't much better. The sellers have been very strategic in their efforts to cover up the warts and wrinkles during the showing. Now that the place is empty, we notice that large holes remain in the floors of several rooms where radiators must have been pulled out years earlier. They'd been covered by rugs before. They've left behind clutter in the closets, garage, and basement. Lots of heavy wood, piles of old paint cans, and rickety furniture that will have to be disposed of.

The backyard is disheartening, not because of the space, but because it has been neglected for longer than I can guess.

Vines and poison ivy hide the small section of chain-link, and the Birch trees, beautiful from the street, are riddled with hollows and branches hang dangerously over the roof and electrical lines. The plumbing has issues and some of the electrical in the basement looks questionable. At least we have a roof over our heads, but this stuff is going to come back to bite us big time. The last thing we need right now is a fixer-upper, but here we are again, forced into a situation with little-to-no option. We can keep storing up problems like this for a while - and we have to, at least until I can get through a transplant, if I ever do - but eventually, we're going to suffer the consequences.

There's not much time to brood over it now. We try to get a hotel but they're all booked due to a No Direction concert at Hershey stadium. The less I say about this the better. We sleep on blow-up mattresses and are saved by the Folson's and our homeschool group the next day when the U-Haul movers flake out. Our new home is full of laughter and friends, people bringing food, kids playing in the yard. It feels like home immediately. I just don't have much time to soak it in because in two months, I start spending two out of every six weeks in the hospital.

Chapter 7

Frequent Flyer

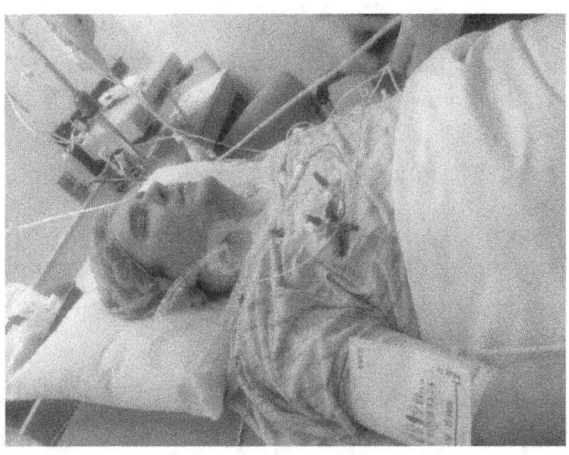

I'm back again, one more year gone by,
I know all the faces, we know what's wrong this time,
Some battles are lost, long before they begin,
It's not surrender, not defeat,
It's just down to sink or swim for your life,
So I'll resign, and launch myself to yellow skies,

Frequent flyer, floating around,
Above the cloud cover, try not to get shot down,
Coasting along, there's no place to land just now,

I'm down again, but I've been here before,
We've seen the crash landings, we know what's in store,
Hellbent but sky-bound, it's a trick of the mind,

I'd rather carry this right now, than leave it all behind,
And say goodbye, just one more time, all to keep myself alight,

Life is good in Pennsylvania. I love the Farmer's Market up the road, our friends, our house (despite the many needed repairs), and I just want things to be normal. The impending swans cath in a few weeks makes me anxious and irritable, and I take it out on everyone around me for weeks prior. Some of the worst fights Christie and I have ever had, usually ending with both of us in tears. I know this is the beginning of yet another long road, unlike the inconvenient and expensive road to St. Louis, or the seemingly eternal road to being listed at Tufts. This will be a road filled with physical pain, isolation, second-guessing, and the temptation of despair and depression.

"It's going to be a war of attrition," Dr. Maron's voice echoes in my head. "Just one small thing after another until, suddenly, you've had enough, and you give up. That's the real danger of this situation."

It's early November and I'm nothing short of impossible to live with. I'm scheduled for my first heart catheterization at Hershey Med Center. But instead of the outpatient procedure I've had before at Tufts in Boston, they'll be leaving the cath in this time, and I'll be living in the hospital with it for an entire week. My last cath procedure at Tufts was grueling, and I'm scared. Terrified, really.

The very first time I'd had this procedure back in the late 90's in Little Rock, I died for a few moments in the recovery area, the "rebound effect," it's called. The nurses brought me back but blamed it on the sedation. At Tufts in 2012, the heart cath was given without sedation.

"It's really not that bad," the technician there had explained. "They numb the spot on the groin where it's inserted and there's some pressure, but people do it without sedation all the time. Better than risking a rebound like you had the last time in Little Rock."

It really was that bad.

A cath procedure is involved, at least for the patient. First, the doctor administers three or four Lidocaine shots around the soft spot of the groin. The needle is long, because the medication needs to go deep into the tissue. Next, a flexible "introducer" - a short, hollow sheath - is inserted into the vein. A wire is then threaded into the sheath to help guide the catheter through the artery all the way into the heart. The doc uses the wire (and sometimes, ultrasound) to advance the cath the entire, winding length of the artery until it reaches the opening to the chambers of the heart - different arteries are used to reach either the right, left, or both. General consensus among patients is that even though it doesn't exactly hurt, it's extremely uncomfortable because you can feel the wire wriggling its way up the inside of your torso into the heart.

That day at Tufts, in 2012, the shots were incredibly painful, and did little to numb the insertion site. The pressure on my groin was tremendous, but I dared not move a millimeter, lest it cause the tech to zig when he should zag. The technician that day wasn't so great at predicting when to zig or zag to begin with. Several times I felt sharp jabs along the way to my heart where he overshot a curve in the artery (my torso ached for days afterward, not to mention the insertion site). To make matters worse, the radio station playing in the lab launched into an hour-long Doors marathon right as the procedure started. I would rather listen to a wailing baby's fingernails on a chalkboard amidst a pack of yipping chihuahuas with the emergency broadcast signal blaring in the background than to listen to even five seconds of any Doors song.

"If there really is a hell," I thought at the time, "this is the damnation sinners will surely suffer there."

Conversations from Room 1170

It was a harrowing experience that made me determined not to do a cath without sedation again. I had no idea what to expect because this time at Hershey, the doc would be entering through the carotid artery on the right side of my neck. Once the wire and cath was in the left chamber of the heart, the part that was still outside of the body would be connected to tubes that could be used to administer medications and draw blood. It would also make it possible for the docs to monitor my cardiac output and pressure ratios in the heart. The line would be stitched or sewn into my neck, with a dressing and tape. It's basically an open passageway to the heart for germs and bacteria, so the site has to be absolutely sealed to prevent infection. The end of the cath that remains on the outside of body would be connected to various machines on an IV pole that would stay by my side for the week. How painful would the whole thing be? The thought of being separated from Christie and the boys for an entire week in a hospital room was the worst torture I could imagine.

The scenario this crisp morning in November replays itself every six weeks over the next two and a half years. We wake to an unseasonably early snowfall. Christie and Rich - twelve at the time - are up before the sun, shoveling the van out of the two-foot snow while it still whitewashes the dawn sky. Brennan and I watch from the windows of the sun room and I wonder again what we were doing, and why. Spending a week apart is counter to everything we've worked for. Aren't we doing all this so we can be together for as long as possible, as much as possible? My odds of surviving HCM are miserable. Maybe I'm wasting my last days with them when I should just accept my fate and enjoy what we have left.

These thoughts ride with me in the passenger seat as Christie navigates the snowy roads. My music of choice on these trips is King's X's "Ear Candy" album. Songs like "Train," "Thinking and Wondering," and "No Room Inside a Box," are like a sedative for my nerves, just as their music has been through this entire experience so far. I alternate between King's X and My Chemical Romance's "The Black Parade" album, a winding musical celebrating the mystery of death and the ripples it causes in the lives of those left behind. Comically morbid, but soothing.

Pennsylvania is, above all, gorgeous in the winter and the stretch from our house down Highway 322 to the med center is rife with quiet dairy farms and endless corn fields. Every corner turned reveals a landscape too beautiful to ever be captured in a picture or painting.

We arrive at the North entrance and Christie drops me and the boys off. She'll have to park in the garage and walk about three-quarters of a mile back to the cath lab waiting room, most of that in the snow this morning, later times in the rain or summer heat. The parking at the hospital, in a word, sucks. The boys stake out a spot near the electric outlets and unpack their laptops and school books. Refusing to stay home or with the Folsons, they'll be there until the procedure is finished and I'm out of the woods, anywhere from three to five o'clock that afternoon.

The needles begin shortly after. My veins are so tiny and shriveled from years of heart failure that no one can get an IV in. It's only needed for sedation, and after the second nurse misses the vein, I consider going without. Someone finally nails the stick, but I'm nauseous by then. This part only gets worse for the next two-and-a-half years.

The boys come to tell me goodbye and we reassure them again that I'll be fine. Of course, Christie and I have no idea if the sedation will cause a rebound again, but I have scores of these procedures ahead of me and we need to find out now.

The transplant coordinator enters my little waiting area where I'm propped up in a stretcher wearing a stereotypically ill-fitting gown. A dark-haired woman in her fifties, she introduces herself and gives us a rundown of how the day will go since it's our first time. She seems pleasant enough until I complain about my scheduled time being pushed back to make way for another patient.

She rounds on me, her eyes blazing, snaps her finger and points at me, interrupting my grumbling with a stern, "No!"

Christie's feathers instantly ruffle. Mine too. We're both thinking it. How dare her. She doesn't know what it's taken to be here, what we've had to do. The sacrifices. About our two boys sitting by themselves, in yet another waiting room, wondering if dad will be okay.

I eventually learn that this woman does

"No!" she repeats continuing to point at me. "This is NOTHING. You think getting bumped is bad? It's going to get So. Much. Worse. than this. So much worse. You start whining about the little things now, how's it going to go when the shit really hits the fan?"

I'm literally agape at this dressing down. Even Christie is speechless. The woman parts the curtain and turns for one more point of the finger and a parting shot, a phrase I will hear dozens of times, that I'll hear for the rest of my life when I encounter hardship.

"Suck it up, buttercup."

Meet Fran Hrenko. Heart transplant coordinator. Whip-cracker. Seer Of All Things. One more person to whom I owe my life.

I don't have to wait long for it to get So. Much. Worse.

The sedation works, mostly. Then it wears off. Then I feel everything.

My neck feels like someone used it for crossbow practice. Throbbing, bruising pain, and a creeping migraine coming on.

They've started the medications (dopamine and dobutamine) at a low drip rate, despite that fact that they're contraindicated for HCM. It's one of the many boxes that have to be checked off for me to meet the UNOS requirements for transplant listing. After the next few visits we realize these drugs are directly to blame for the migraines and the nausea, but little can be done about it. Gotta check the box. Thankfully, over time we notice that the drugs actually did actually reduce my ever-present fluid around the lungs - always a danger because once the fluid volume becomes too great, it can enter the lungs and drown you from the inside.

It takes hours to get a room, and nearly that long to get Tylenol, the only pain med I'm allowed at that time. When they do finally wheel me into the HVIC, it's into a rather cozy, private room with a sliding glass door, bathroom, and recliner. I can't say that I felt at home in those early days, but I fell in love with the nursing staff immediately.

I always hear voices and see faces when coming out of sedation, but I'm not generally lucid until about the time I get to the HVI room. And Natalie, just as she was that first time, is always there to meet me. Once I've seen Christie and the boys, hers is the first face I look for. She is slight, with cropped blond hair, and a quiet confidence. Always ready with Tylenol, water, extra pillows, and a persistent strength that along with Christie's, carry me through those first awful hours. She is the main reason I believe I'm in the right place for a heart transplant, as so much depends on the nursing staff post-procedure.

At shift change, Jenn, the night shift nurse, older, confident, gentle but commanding, takes her place until morning. By nothing more than a coincidence of scheduling, I'm fortunate enough to have these two for my admissions the first six or eight times in a row.

The first night is always a blur of neck pain, back pain, sweating, thirst, and headache. Christie is up all night with me while the boys stay with the Folsons. I don't truly come back to myself until morning. The sedation has worn off, the pain in my neck has subsided a bit, and I'm in my right mind. Or as right as my mind can be. Christie, awake now for over twenty-four hours, feels confident enough in my mental faculties and the nursing staff to leave me and get some sleep. She's worked five, twelve-hour shifts in a row so she can be off this week. This allows her to be off the first night I'll be back home so she can keep an eye on the cath site (the cath now removed) because the blood clot that forms when it's taken out can sometimes burst. You don't want to bleed to death from your carotid or femoral artery in your sleep. But this meant she'd have to work three shifts in a row after that. Added up - every time I have a swans cath and a two-week hospital stay, we are all apart for roughly fifteen consecutive days (save my first night how). This is our routine, about twenty-four times over the next year and a half.

After the first night, I face the week. First, getting from the bed to the chair, then finally to the bathroom. Then onto the HVI unit to walk laps, dragging my IV pole with me (I affectionately name him "Dr. Dooda"), nurse following behind.

Through conversations with Fran and the docs, we realize that they intend for me to do this every month or so.

"About every six or seven weeks we'll bring you in and do this," Fran tells me. "That way we keep up with what's happening, and you get some 1A time. Maybe a heart will come for you while you're here. Never know."

More likely than it would have been a year ago. Several transplant programs, including Hershey, have instituted an "O for O" policy in which O+ blood type hearts are first offered to O+ blood type candidates, rather than to the entire pool of candidates regardless of blood type (remember that while anyone can take an O+ heart, O+ blood types can only take an O+ heart). It will still be an unpredictably long wait, but regardless, we'll be planning our lives around these hospital stays for the foreseeable future (months? Years?). It was ridiculously difficult to plan for this one alone, between Christie's work schedule, and someone to watch the boys (which the Folsons do at first). Blitzy and the Folson's dog, Scout don't mix well, so she has to stay at home, but no dog can be left for too long without going outside. Christie's shift is twelve hours, and she tries to catch the doctors during rounds in the morning before going home. Not to mention, she has to start back to school for her bachelor's degree as per her contract with Penn State. How is all of this going to work? It's too much to even think about and Christie leaves that first morning distraught and overwhelmed. It doesn't help that a friend tells her later that day, "Well, this is your life now. You should be used to it."

My concerns are more immediate - the food is terrible, beyond terrible, especially given my recent foray into gourmet cooking at home. I learn to ask for meal vouchers instead, and Christie brings marginally better food from the cafeteria. She uses FMLA and PTO time to be with me or bring the boys up on some days near the beginning of all this. After being together 24/7 on the road and at home for the last few years, the parting of ways on these nights is excruciating more than any physical pain I experience during my admissions. I stand at the double doors leading away from the HVI, playing stupid peek-a-boo games with the boys as they leave. They're way too old for this, which is what makes it so funny, but eventually I disappear for the last time around the corner. Christie needs to get them home. I have no idea how long they ever waited there to see if I'd pop back out again. The walk back to the room seems very long on those nights. I usually stop and sit for a while in the big wide window sill that overlooks the ground and north parking lot. Dr. Dooda and I make a few laps and go to bed.

***

One admission blurs into the next, me running around like a crazy person in between trying to make small home repairs, spend time with friends, and hang out with the boys. The Folsons have introduced us to a new world of modern board-gaming, with which we become a bit obsessed. Each new admission finds us huddled around a card table in the small hospital room, eating shrimp pasta or meatloaf that Christie's brought to leave with me, then playing an hours long game of Settlers of Catan, Ticket to Ride, Carkasonne, Candamere, High Noon Saloon, or Tiki Mountain. The doctors and nurses chuckle and shake their heads.

"It's our living room," Christie tells them. "He can't come to his, so we bring it here." And she does, consistently, for nearly three years. It keeps me sane.

We're hunched over a particularly complex Settlers of Catan expansion one afternoon when a couple appears in the doorway.

"You're Dave," the burly, bearded guy says. He's older than me and has a jolly smile that makes St. Nick look like a perpetrator. There's something mischievous there too. His wife beams at the boys.

"Yeah?"

"Mudge," he says, and extends his hand. "My wife, Terri. You have HCM."

"I do!" As rare as it is to meet doctors who know the disease well enough to call it that, meeting a patient that knows it is even more rare.

"Same. I'm waiting on a heart too."

We're all stunned. Up until this point, I figure I'm the only person on the planet waiting for a heart transplant because of HCM. I know they exist, but here one was, live and in the flesh.

"I've been here for two weeks, headed home," he says.

"I live here," I joke. His laugh also puts St. Nick to shame. Jolly doesn't cover it. It's deep and infectious. This guy has a story, I tell myself.

"Yep. You're a frequent flyer. Like me. There are a few of us."

"Frequent flyer?" Brennan asks.

"That's what they call us around here. Racking up the miles. Hopefully we get to cash them in soon, huh?"

Hopefully the whole damn plane doesn't crash, I think to myself. But he's right. Always in a holding pattern. Never knowing what's happening on the ground, or what's going on in the cockpit. No place to land at the moment. And the gas tank is getting dry.

Mudgeman is a fixture on the HVI; he's been coming in with swans catheters to accumulate "1A" time for two years. He would soon become a fixture in our lives, and he and his wife Terri remain so as of this writing.

He has to come for 1A time, just like me. At home, we're low men on the totem pole as far as the UNOS list goes. When we're admitted on IV drugs, we bank precious "IA" time, buying us a higher status on the list for those days of admission. It's even possible we could get the call while admitted, an impossibility at home. Mudge and I pass through each other's lives from time to time, but we both take solace in knowing we're not alone in the vast wasteland of HCM transplant-dom.

Other things happen over time. A friendship develops between our family and Dr. Eric Popjes, the cardiologist for whom we moved to Hershey. He is in fact, an incredible resource for an HCM info-junkie like me. He's also a Star Wars nerd, eliciting immediate trust from yours truly. True, old-school, dark-age surviving Star Wars fans will understand this, and I won't bore you with it here. But that instinct has never disappointed me.

I begin to tolerate the procedure, sometimes without sedation, especially when hot-shot cardiologist, Dr. Boehmer is in the cockpit. I generally arrive in my room alert and ready to get the two weeks over with. Bank the time, get to the top of the list, get this over with. But I have to do the time. We quote the old

Hindu saying a lot: "How do you eat an elephant? One bite at a time."

Fran becomes not only a confidant, but a protector, a pit-bull on my behalf, and the bearer of hard truths. She nor Popjes pull punches when discussing the bleak reality of my situation. And it's a comfort after so much corporatism and slush from St. Louis and feeling a bit lost in the shuffle once we settled in at Tufts in Boston. At one point in the middle of this long stretch, I begin to worry a lot, because my cath procedures are being postponed, and I've even been sent home without the procedure once. Bed space is high-dollar real estate in the Hershey HVI and I'm often rescheduled because there simply isn't room for me. This starts to eat at me. I've been dumped or abandoned by two programs at this point and the feeling is unsettlingly familiar. I spill my guts to Fran on the phone in a torrent of worry and frustration one afternoon.

"You're right," she says after she absorbs everything. "If this is the plan - the admissions, the swans, the 1A time, then it needs to be a priority for us. I'm going to bring this to the group in our Tuesday meeting. You listen to me, kid. We're not dumping you. I don't dump people. I told you we're getting you a heart, and that's how this is going to go. I know it's dark right now, and it's going to get even darker by the time we're through. I've promised you that. But we're going to get through it, together, you and I. You remember this conversation because we're going to be laughing about it at your one-year post-biopsy." I have no choice but to trust her. I'm less confident that there will ever be a one-year biopsy.

We finally and fully introduce the boys to Firefly, the one-season space western directed by Joss Whedon in the mid 00's that Fox deliberately sabotaged into cancellation. I know – it seems trivial to even mention a television show in a story like this, but the story of the Firefly crew becomes our story in so many ways throughout all of this. A group of misfit scavengers on the outskirts of barely settled space, trying to get by anyway they can.

Pay your dues, get the payoff, keep flying. Same for us. Do the thing. Do the time. Stay airborne. Frequent Flyers. Captain Mal Reynolds is fighting a losing battle, and everyone around him knows it. But through sheer determination and reckless spite, he always comes out on the other side, bruised, burnt, broke, but alive. His beleaguered troops face hopeless odds in the first episode, a situation met with Mal's optimistic assertion that, "We've done the impossible, and that makes us mighty." These words become scripture to us.

***

Another Valentine's day, 2014. I'm in and out of lucidity, trying to wake up fully from the Dilaudid in my system. In those early days, Christie left the recovery suite to walk across the campus and stand outside, rain, snow, or heat, to get a cellphone signal and update our parents on my condition. After missing important info about my numbers one time, and a vomit inducing mistake with the inotropic drugs another, she couldn't do it anymore. At first, she'd call the Folsons who sent out an email to spread the word, but eventually, our friend Ellen Gecker (gracious wife of our realtor, Marc) starts coming to the hospital to make the calls so Christie can stay with me. Why such a large hospital and college campus has such terrible cell service is beyond me. They have enough money to buy Verizon or Sprint outright. It's a constant frustration on days like these, trying to communicate with family, or the boys in the rare instance that they aren't with us.

The urgent knock-knock on my bladder wall renders me semi-alert. Squinting without my glasses, I realize I'm on a Bumex drip – a strong diuretic, especially when given through an IV. I have Bill as my nurse for the first time. Bill botched my IV placement twice before calling another nurse to do it, so I'm already not impressed by Bill. He's probably unaware of my desire to crush him with the arm that wasn't stabbed three times earlier. I desperately search around for something to pee in and spot a blurry, white, urinal-shaped blob on the shelf near the door.

I hit the call light as every inch of my excretory system does acrobatics to keep from wetting myself. Bumex is insistent - if you can't find a bathroom, you'd better find a Depends because the urine is exiting your body no matter how much you try to hold it back.

The button doesn't light up, and I hear nothing but silence from the desk, so even if the light is broken, there's no call bell going off up front. I give it another hard push and realize the cord is way too long. Because it's not even plugged in.

I try to use The Force to levitate the urinal to my bed, but I'm not yet far enough along in my Jedi training to have mastered the skill. Or to hold back the call of The Force itself on my bladder.

I start yelling for help, but no one comes. I decide to just get up and get the urinal myself; very ill-advised. The nurses reading this are yelling, "NO," out loud at this point because no one wants An Incident. A sedated patient, hooked up to an IV pole, lurching around the room, always leads to An Incident. And not the "oopsie, I'm dizzy, let me sit down for a moment" kind of Incident. More the kind of Incident that involves falling into the sharp corners of furniture and cabinets, head injuries, trauma, and a thesis paper worth of forms to fill out and file. In my delirium, not peeing the bed is for some reason more of a threat to my personal safety.

But that won't work either. Bill has both bed rails up and in the locked position for this flight. No paperwork on his watch. Guess he'd rather clean up urine.

My attempts to climb over the railing finally sets off a bed alarm. Elizabeth, who I called Grumpy Nurse at the time, runs in, catches a full moon since my gown is hiked up past my knees in my escape attempt, and yells at me for trying to leave the bed.

Doing my best Cheech and/or Chong impression, I explain to her that I need the urinal, the call bell is unplugged, and that something's wrong with The Force in this room. She plugs in the alarm, shoves the urinal at me and runs back to her patients. Where is Bill? I barely have time to ponder this because I'm asleep again still holding the now-warm 900 cc urinal in my hand. It's full to the 700-cc mark.

I awake to Bill's gruff apology, then watch from the bed in horrified, drug-induced stupor as four men in tuxedos, red bow ties, and cumber buns sing Let Me Call You Sweetheart in slamming barbershop harmonies. They launch into Paper Moon and I decide if I'm going to hallucinate, I may as well enjoy the ride. I sing along at the top of my lungs. Hallucination or no, I'm not missing a chance to sing a Sinatra jag. We're ripping into the bridge with feeling ("Without your love...it's a honky tonk parade, without your love...it's a melody played in a penny arcade!" My God, Frank had swagger to spare...) when a sports car like something from a kiddie ride at the fair pulls up in the doorway.

I've never been stoned before - this must be what everyone was on about in high school. Way more fun than I ever imagined. I almost forget the searing pain in my neck.

The tenor is fantastic. I get their card. "I've always wanted to sing barbershop," I tell him. "When all this is done, I'm going to find you guys and we're gonna sing."

They pat my arm and wish me well. In the full presence of the gaggle of nurses who've gathered around my bed to listen, they wish me, "Happy Valentine's Day. From Matt." They reward my puzzled expression with a teddy bear and an M&M filled heart. The rumors persist to this day.

The drugs, it turns out, aren't really that good. The sports car was a portable X-Ray borrowed from pediatrics. The quartet was intended for Christie and me, a Valentine gift from the Folsons (though Matt's name alone made it onto the card).

But where is Christie? She took the boys home but is usually back by now to spend the first night with me. I'm worried, because this is a pattern I've discouraged to no avail. All her vacation days and FMLA used up, she works a twelve-hour shift, drives home to shower, drives the four of us back to the hospital for the cath procedure, stays for the duration, takes the boys home and gets them settled, then returns to the hospital to spend the night. Most of the time, she's been awake a full 46 plus hours by the time she crashes in the uncomfortable, non-reclining recliner in the room, and is woken constantly by nurses taking my vitals every two hours and me moaning and groaning in between.

She finally calls the desk from the van, hissing out words through clenched teeth.

"I have a kidney stone, maybe a cyst," she tells one of the nurses. "Tell Dave I'm going to the ER." Not unthinkable. She fought her own war with life-threatening endometriosis and ovarian cysts when we were in high school and newly married.

She arrives, limping, into my room around 3 a.m. It was a kidney stone, but it's more. There is a big spot on her gallbladder, which is either infected … or a mass. The ER doc wants a biopsy, as soon as possible. He worries it's cancer.

Now what? She can't have the procedure until I'm out, so she schedules it for the earliest date possible. This situation dominates our conversation the remainder of my stay. How to deal with cancer on top of everything else...we don't say it but we both know this could very possibly be where the wheels start coming off the bus. Our finances, our parenting...our sanity. It's a long week and when the day comes, the biopsy shows nothing abnormal. Christie juggles nights off with co-workers to get the time off to rehabilitate. The time at home is nice, but we're both down and out. The boys pick up the slack again.

This frequent flying blurs into monotony for two and a half years. Eventually, Fran convinces us to do two weeks at a time instead of one. Our decision to go ahead with it is based on the wild hope that I'll get the call while I'm there. I was number three on the list during my most recent admission, and Fran thinks we're close. I hope so. I'm retaining fluid quicker than the meds can get rid of it. My weight is up to 228, an estimated 25 pounds of that, water retention. Extreme temperatures are becoming intolerable, and I can barely make the staircase up to our bedroom at night.

In the midst of all this, we learn from Mudgeman's wife, Terri, that he's been transplanted. She says that he got the call just as he was packing to go home at the end of his two-week admission and had a raging fit at Dr. Boehmer because he wanted to forfeit his place on the list to me. I barely know the guy, but I remember he and his wife Terri in tears the last time they saw us sitting around the card table in my room, eating dinner together. She told me she didn't think they could have done this with young kids. Nevertheless, we're exuberantly happy for him. The news of an HCM patient actually being transplanted is a win for everyone, and word gets around quick in our small community.

By this time, Christie's FMLA and PTO days are long gone. We're surviving my admissions on vacation days, call-ins resulting in lost wages, and co-worker donated personal time. It becomes laborious and complicated to have the boys stay with the Folsons every time I'm admitted, and we can tell the monotony is wearing them thin as well. A homeschool teenage friend agrees to stay nights with the boys for way cheaper than she should have while Christie works. This way, the dog is taken care of, the boys aren't displaced, and we're not spread apart as a family between four locations all the time. It works much better for us, but the Folsons take it as a slight, and we sense a distance growing in the relationship. The kids are growing apart too, and just as we warned them (and anyone who offers us help), it's become a one-sided relationship, us doing all the taking, never the giving. We try, but we fail often. We confess it openly, and often, because we know the burden it must be to expose yourself to such a dismal situation constantly, with no promises, end, or positive outcome in sight. We learn to let people go and not be angry at them. I can't say I would persist in such a situation if I had the choice to leave, or simply fade away.

Other homeschool friends take up the slack, Jenn McCurdy, and the ever-present reformed hippies, Marc and Ellen Gecker, our realtor and his wife. Marc and I spend time talking and messing about on our guitars between admissions, watching old Marx Brothers films, 60's rock documentaries, and eating take-out. The boys take to them like grandparents, and they can often be found at a baseball game or mini-golf course together. The relationship is bittersweet to Christie and I who realize the boys can't do any of this with their own grandparents, so far away in Arkansas. But we're grateful they have older people in their lives, and Marc is a character bursting with joy and hope, in awe of their creativity, and always introducing them to new things, be it the stock market, or old Janis Joplin performances. As unlucky as we are to be so far from grandparents, Marc and Ellen come into our lives, and more importantly into the boys lives at the exact right moment in time. Their conversations with Ellen about life, death, and the unknown are probably the most valuable they'll have with anyone through this period of time. She listens without judgement or opinion, and they in turn feel safe with her because she gets it - she lost her own mother to illness at a young age and it disrupted her life completely. I feel the same with Marc, and neither of them have expectations of us. They intuitively understand our strong desire to keep things as normal as possible for the boys and conform to that without explanation or resistance. It's refreshing and scary all at once.

Songs start pouring out of me. I've written a few since we left Arkansas, but now it's like a flood. I don't bring my guitar with me to the hospital, but I have recording software on my computer. Over the course of six months, I write an entire album via humming into my computer mic and programming the bass, drums, strings, piano, and other instruments with sequencers and samples. It becomes the framework for my Instead of Wither album, a concept work about my struggle with faith and decision to leave the ministry. I have no idea why this issue, resolved, rears its ugly head now, but I just go where it takes me. Between admissions, I'm in the basement in a makeshift vocal booth with a cheap microphone recording live guitars and vocals. My decade long obsession with The Beatles pays off; I can hear the Lennon/McCartney influence in the songs, and even Harrison creeping in from time to time. I think they're the strongest songs I've ever written, especially lyrically, and I now feel a rush to finish the project as soon as I can, in case the worst happens soon. It's a story I needed to tell, so I won't recount it here; you have to buy the album for that one (shameless plug…).

I get progressively comfortable with my surroundings with each cath procedure and admission. The names of the cath lab team, the nurses, the doctors. I learn their schedules and slide easily into the ebb and flow of life on the unit.

The first time I don't have a bed awaiting on the HVI, I'm with Rick all night. The day shift starts clearing out, and he's new, unsure, and completely freaked out to have an HCM patient on inotrope drips that are contraindicated. I'm asking for pain meds and for the drips to be titrated down. He wrings his hands a lot, hoping for help from the others who are busy with other patients. It's a skeleton crew anyway, that time of night, and Rick's afraid to do anything because HCM patients are infamous for having adverse reactions to sudden changes in meds or fluids. He watches over me like a mother hen that night, and what begins as an antagonistic relationship, blooms into respect as we work through the various issues I'm having together. He gets me through the night safely and finally into a room in the early morning hours. Rick ends up being my pre and post cath nurse for almost all of my future procedures, even changing his schedule to be there for me if I'm on the list. Bill and Elizabeth, a.k.a. Grumpy Nurse, become equally protective of me in time, especially once they realize how often I'm here, and I develop a deep trust in them both.

We figured it would continue this way until either I died or got the call. But despite our rigorous "what if" lists and considering all the variables, something, and someone, blindsided us. We weren't prepared for either, but I'd be dead without them both.

Chapter 8

Rite as Reign

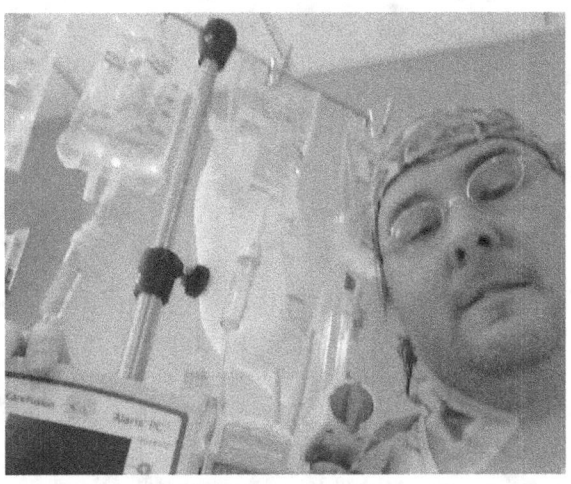

The banks are flooded, the downpour taken hold,
Filling basements wrecking lawns, the river overflows,
I'm feeling fine, I could swim my way right out of here,
Hold my breath, throw me a line, and a remedy for fear,

I'm right as rain, this pain is just an illusion,
I'm right as rain, sorry for the confusion,

Good sense is drowned, the weather man finally gets the ax,
It's pelting cats and dogs, I can last forever on my back,
Fashionistas with umbrellas shout advice from the wall,
It's hard to hear over this waterfall

Jesus, can you take the time, to throw a drowning man a line,
Is this some kind of test down here?
Cause I can't tell the lesson from the drowning,
The current has me by the tail,
third time under, too far from the rail,
One more chance to win or fail

Chronic illness isn't what you think. It does more damage from the inside out than the outside in; crippling, maiming, debilitating, disfiguring. It requires pills that do things to your body and mind than are harder to live with than the original problem. Thing is, the side effects from those chemicals won't actually kill you. The thing you're taking them for will. It's not even the lesser of the evils - it's just one more thing the sickness inflicts on you. Be even sicker, so that you don't get so sick that you die.

We know what disease looks like. You can spot it easily in a crowd because it's an aberration - it stands out. It's the old man in the motorized grocery cart, caregiver with oxygen tank in tow. It's the crumpled-up kid in the wheelchair, the bald woman in line at the bank. It simultaneously evokes shock and empathy (for those of us who aren't health insurance CEO's or Big Pharma shareholders – you know, actual humans). We can see the effect their disease has on them - it's right there, in living color before us, struggling to make it back to the handicapped spot or up the stairs. Rightly so, we open doors for them, let them go first, have an extra measure of patience when they are slow to order, or pay, or try to scuttle out of the way so as not to inconvenience the "normal" people. They're usually grateful, and seldom need to ask for these things, because the reason for this disparity between themselves and healthy people is evident to all.

The world doesn't work that way for folks with invisible illnesses. My first experience was thirty seconds after I'd been diagnosed with Hypertrophic Cardiomyopathy and given no explanation of exactly what that was. I was twenty-eight years old and Dr. Santoro of the Baptist Hospital Cardiac Group in Little Rock, Arkansas (yes, I'm naming names), cut his eyes suspiciously at me when I asked blankly if it was safe for me to work. I was a musician, and looked like one at the time, long hair in braids, unruly beard, assorted jewelry clanking around on my arms and around my neck. He looked me up and down with derision, scoffed and asked, "Do you even work?" I chose a different cardiologist within the week and never paid the bill. I owned a floor servicing company at the time and worked harder in a single night that he'd worked in his entire life, judging from his hands.

I didn't look sick, and he thought it was ridiculous that I felt sick - even a cardiologist. That dynamic intensified as my HCM progressed. Invisible illnesses that are also chronic, wreak the same destruction, but they do something more insidious than physical damage. They destroy your personality, your self-confidence, and your dignity.

When I first started having to announce to business partners and band mates that I had been diagnosed with a fatal heart disease, they were largely incredulous.

"You just played a two-hour gig last weekend!"

"You look better than ever, man. You just carried all those 5 gallons in from the truck."

"Eh, sometimes doctors get things wrong. Don't let 'em scare you. You look fine."

Where this ridiculous notion that a person who looks fine must also feel fine comes from, I have no idea. I learned early on that the first rule of HCM is; how you look, and even sometimes how you feel are irrelevant. This is why HCM is often associated with sudden cardiac death (SCD) in young athletes. The picture of health on the outside, deadly mitral valve obstruction and arrhythmias on the inside. It's why high school basketball players and even an Olympic runner ("FloJo") fall dead in the middle of practice.

Curiously, my college Bible study kids got it right away, back in 1998. They jumped to work, learned the floor business from Christie, taking over jobs, even following me to the ones they couldn't do just to unload and re-load the equipment. I looked the same to them, but they knew something wasn't right in my manner, my spirit, that my essential "Dave-ness" was being drained. The four that we had grown closest to, Leslie, Jason, Tiffany, and Spencer even took to bending down to tie my shoes for me. So did Robin, our house-mate at the time. They learned the things that had suddenly become hard for me to do, the things that knocked my wind out or left me pale.

But those kids were seniors. They graduated and moved away for the most part, and I was the pastor of a church that didn't really grasp the situation. I constantly had to insist that I couldn't take care of the roofing debris in the winter cold or be present at every single church event. Why I sat out of the worship team some days. Though our lives seemed to eventually return to "normal" about a year after my diagnosis, it had changed dramatically. I had changed dramatically.

And so it has gone, year after year.

Yelled at for parking in a handicapped space.

Called lazy for not helping lift a 350 lb. woman in a wheelchair down the front steps of an apartment building during a fire alarm.

Told by security not to sit on the floor at a standing room only event.

Told I should get a job. Go to college. Exercise more. Eat better. Pray harder. Think more positively.

Things that would never have happened had there been some outward evidence of my HCM. I know this because I've gone on to use canes, walkers, and other external devices and was finally treated like a sick person. A simple cane is a miracle stick. Even a limp following a femoral catheter does the trick. I wonder if there's a way to sneak Dr. Doo-da (my IV pole) out of the hospital so I can drag him around with me everywhere I go. Seeing is believing, right?

Invisible illnesses steal who you are. You begin to see yourself as others do. You begin to think of yourself as the lazy, dependent, labor-dodging bum that strangers assume you are. You become more and more reliant on others, and you see yourself at times as an idiot child, taken by the hand and led where you must go, for your own good, because you can't do it for yourself.

But oh, how you'll try. I hate so much having to explain to other men that I can't help put the tables away, or stack the chairs, or help them move, that I'll go ahead and muscle through it anyway. I'm sick for days afterwards, but at least they didn't think I was lazy. Because my disease convinces me sometimes that I am.

The beta-blockers and calcium channel blockers have started playing tricks with my short-term memory now. I can't keep up with my car keys, but it doesn't matter anymore, because I get lost when I drive. I'm constantly missing appointments or commitments, constantly second guessing if I remember the time correctly. Everyone around me, including the boys, are managing a toddler. Except that I get frustrated and tired of being babied and lash out when they take it upon themselves to do things for me that I have the illusion I can do for myself. I've lost confidence in my ability to form coherent arguments, to discern fatigue from apathy.

The worst part of this is when friends who are close begin to find humor in it, and not the loving, good natured, "let's get through this together," kind of humor. Rather, the eye-rolling, exasperated put-upon humor that is nothing more than thinly veiled resentment. As I deteriorate, I find some of our homeschool friends treating me with suspicion when I ask someone to pick the boys up for the park or an activity (even though they've offered repeatedly). We start to catch wind of the sentiment that I'm not really as sick as I'm making out - that I'm playing it up for sympathy and favors. I long so badly to be at the park with my boys, at the pool, playing lazer tag and riding go-carts. Instead, I'm home on the couch, white-knuckling my way through yet another bout of A-fib, or angina, or sleeping off a cardioversion or swans catheter sedation.

But you start to believe these things of yourself. Maybe I am playing it up. Maybe it's worse in my head than it is in reality. Maybe I like staying home, while other people chauffeur my kids around. Maybe I'm just a bad parent. I'm aware of how short a step it is from that thought to the more dangerous one; why am I sticking around anyway? I know HCM patients who have put guns in their mouths because they took that last, deadly step.

It only takes a gun to blow it all away

***

It's the fall of 2014. I've been a Frequent Flyer for over a year now and I can't think clearly about these things anymore. I feel like a laughingstock, the man-child who must be kept and watched at all times lest he hurt himself or forget some crucial detail. Christie tries valiantly to let me maintain what independence I have left, but I fail at nearly every opportunity to remember, to stay up to speed, to take care of it on my own, whatever "it" is.

If only I had a scar to show, or a cane to walk on. I could prove to them all that this isn't really me. I ran a successful business, for god sakes, built it from the ground up. Formed, recorded albums with, and toured with half-a-dozen bands playing various instruments. I ran a 300-man Dad's volunteer program. I pastored a church that still stands to this day. I've written three books, co-created an internationally acclaimed PC game mod, recorded three albums worth of music nearly on my own, raised and homeschooled two kids, and taught myself to cook like a chef.

"This is not me!" I want to scream. "All you can see is the shadow of who I used to be."

Chances are slim that I'll ever be that person again. Maybe my mind is permanently damaged beyond being able to recover the sharpness I once had. Maybe I'll never have the confidence to do anything again. For the people in my life now, here, in Pennsylvania, in this moment in time, this is the only Dave they know. I hate it, and I hate him for being so frail and unsure of himself. I am beyond rescue from myself, and I even resort to prayer, something I'd abandoned years earlier. As always, I receive no reply, no warm rush of blood, no supernatural or material evidence that I'm doing anything other than talking out loud to myself. I figure that's the next step in my mental unwinding anyway.

I'm sorry for Christie and the boys. They've watched me deteriorate into this shell of a person. The boys will never remember me as musician Dad, pastor Dad, Watchdog Dad, or business owner Dad. I've become sitting-in-the-recliner hallucinating from Percocet between fits of wakeful sleep Dad.

But I restrain myself from telling anyone these things except Christie. There's no need - she's the eyewitness to it. Everyone offers advice, from the safety and comfort of their effortlessly healthy lives. I can barely focus on conversations anymore, much less take their advice seriously. I'm drowning, but I'll keep telling everyone I'm okay, I'm hanging in there. Because I wouldn't want the things I've said here dumped on me if the shoe was on the other foot. Not over and over. It's not what anyone wants to hear and I can't take the looks of pity or concerned grimaces most days. I just want to stay away from everyone and pretend I'm someone else.

Why am I even still here?

Chapter 9

Indestructible

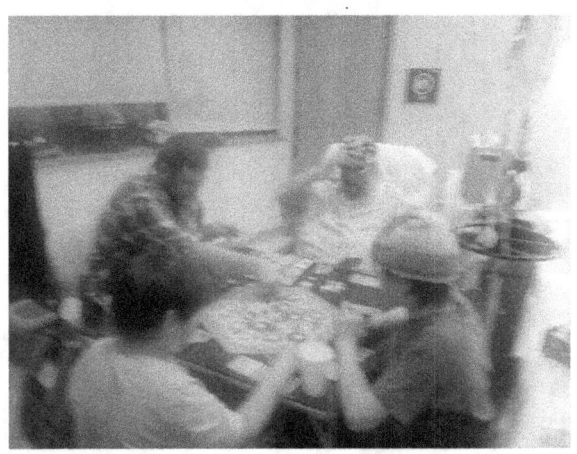

He was living in the future, breaking all the rules,
Reigning over empires full of simpletons and fools,
Walking laps around the world in the middle of the night,
The waiting and the burning down, the honor and the spite,

And we knew we shouldn't say it,
We knew that it was only for today,
But we knew just how to play it,
Dreams lose out to breathing, and no one gets away

When the house of cards comes crashing down,
And the King of the Hill throws down his crown,
Fear and courage look the same, and everyone was fooled,
Was it a crime for me to think, you were indestructible?

Conversations from Room 1170

We were standing in the balance, of faith and unbelief,
Years kept blurring past him, childhood was a thief,
He said, "the ending makes no difference,
it's how you run the race,"
The only way to beat it down is to stare it in the face

And we knew we shouldn't tempt it,
We knew that it was coming for us all,
We knew we'd never lift it,
I cannot raise my voice to scream,
now there's a flatline down the hall,

I can't get it out of my head,
They cut him up and everybody bled,
I can't hear what they're telling me,
it's all bouncing off the walls,
I don't care what anyone says, you were indestructible

"There it is again," I whisper to Christie, but she's deep in sleep, propped once again in the torturous recliner in the corner. Maybe the lingering sedation is playing tricks on my ears.

Wish-woosh, wish woosh, WWish whoosh, WISH, WHOOSH, Wish whoosh, wish whoosh.

A rhythmic sloshing, dry clicking sound that Dopplers in from down the hall, passes the door to my room, then Dopplers away as it passes. It's been doing it on and off for hours this first night of my two-week stay. It's December of 2015 and I've never heard that dry sound from a floor scrubber. I finally drift off, remembering the many nights I piloted such a machine in the bowels of some office building, hospital, or grocery store. I hated it at the time, but I'd give anything to be pushing one tonight, The Statler Brothers or Slayer blaring away in my headphones instead of here in bed getting to know my twenty-something-th swans catheter.

Dr. Clemens did the honors, and I was very clear (in good humor) with him after, that it is not his gift. His insertion point is so high on my neck that the bandage actually covers part of my ear and sticks in my hair. To make matters worse, I've developed a nasty skin allergy to the bandage adhesive and start developing blisters within a few days after the procedure. Blisters can cause the white blood cell count to rise -which gets checked every day - and if it's elevated, the cath gets pulled and I get sent home, losing valuable 1A time. The burning itch gets worse each day until they either send me home, or I've fiddled with it so much, the bandage has to be replaced. The skin is raw underneath, so the Chlorohexidine cleanings that accompany a bandage change are agonizing.

We've lost all access to the heart from the right side of my neck over the fall, so now they're going in from the left. "Occluded," is the term. But even that's getting dicey, and the docs are having to do some very creative placement to make it go down at all. No more swans caths, no more IA time, down to sitting at home, floating at the bottom of the list again, wasting away.

The next day, I sit in my recliner, now pulled next to the sliding door so I have a view of the unit, headphones on, working on bass and string arrangements for what will become my fourth album Instead of Wither. I don't look up much until during a pause to a reboot, and I hear the swishing noise again.

He can't be more than eighteen, a short-ish, stocky kid with that awkward post-pubescent growth of beard. He tromps past my room, his face a cloud of indifference. The noise comes from a backpack he's wearing. Some new LVAD (left ventricular assist device)?

I don't even think much about the backpack. I'm riveted by his clothing. He's wearing an Ohio football jersey and saggy cargo shorts, and street shoes with actual socks. Not those scratchy yellow hospital things, either. Real socks.

Fran tells me later that afternoon that I need to meet him.

"Oh, Perry?" she asks with a knowing grin. "That's quite a story. You should pop in and say hi to him while you're here."

Fran is always working an angle, so I suspect that she set the whole thing up. I wouldn't be surprised to learn that she'd had the HVI switch patients around to put Perry and I on the same side of the unit so that his incessant lapping of the halls would bring him past my door repeatedly.

He stops once and gruffly introduces himself. I stop him in the hall a few days later to invite him to eat with us that night. He says he will but doesn't. This goes back and forth several times the first week.

I notice that he's developed quite a camaraderie with Tommy, Shaun, Adam, and a bunch of the male nurses. I hear them joking around late into the night while I try unsuccessfully to sleep on my back. Still, after almost two years, I'm not used to it.

I learn bits and pieces from the nurses - he's fine with them talking about his situation. He was admitted directly from the pediatric ward the minute he turned eighteen. HCM patient, and they actually had to take his entire heart out and replace it with a total artificial one - a T(otal) A(rtificial) H(eart) - TAH, it was called. The backpack carries the pump that powers the heart. He's been fighting HCM as a patient of Dr. Popjes since he was seven years old. Everyone loves him.

"How?" I wonder. He's kind of a jerk. He's not friendly, he doesn't talk, and we've tried to invite him to eat...maybe he's just really private.

Christie can't stand it. She finally tracks him down one afternoon, tempting him with garlic chicken and cabbage, an actual home-cooked meal. He grudgingly arrives at my room, backpack in tow, and digs in without saying much. Which just isn't possible - you know, if you've ever had Christie's garlic chicken and cabbage.

"Oh my God, this is incredible," he says after a few mouthfuls. "It's so good. You made this?" It occurs to me that he's been eating hospital food for some time.

"How long have you been in this time?" I ask.

"Six months," he says, shoveling another fork-full.

My time as a pastor has trained me to give nothing away by my facial expression, but that training fails me miserably at this revelation.

"Six MONTHS?"

"Have to," he says, motioning to the backpack on the floor. "Went home for a while but had to come back. Machine kept acting up. I was here most of last year, on the peds ward." He says all of this like we're discussing a video game, one we're not very passionate about.

The backpack emits a series of loud beeps, which scares the beJezus out of the four of us. He seems not to notice, takes a few more bites, then grabs up the backpack and hustles out the door.

"Be right back - is there more of that?" He points to the chicken, still chewing.

"Yes sir," Christie laughs. "I brought extra for Dave, but he won't eat it all, so you can have some of it."

"Oh…" He seems puzzled by her generosity. "Ok, thanks. Be right back."

I don't remember our hurried conversation while he was gone those few minutes, but I'm sure it was along the lines of, "and we think we're going through a tough time because we do this two WEEKS at a time? Maybe we should shut-up more."

He re-enters with a power chord which he plugs into the wall and sticks the other end into a jack on the side of the backpack. A torrent of questions follow.

"How long does the battery last?"

"So, it's like a TOTAL artificial heart? So you don't actually have a human heart right now? As I'm talking to you. No heart."

"What happens if the batteries run out?"

"How long can you survive on one of those?"

At least, I'm sure the kids asked all of this. I'm fixated on the fact that the guy has a plastic heart sewn into his chest, and he's sitting here eating without getting winded. He's been lapping this HVI unit - 88 steps in a lap (I know because, well, you'll see) - like mad for the last week. He went outside to shoot hoops with Tommy and Sean yesterday.

He's healthier than I am.

Out comes Settlers of Catan, our go-to game when playing "our" board games with someone new.

I should take a moment to explain "our" board games. A Renaissance has taken place in the board game industry in the last ten years or so. It started in 1995 with the English version of a German made game called . . .The Settlers of Catan. As of this writing, it's approaching twenty-three million copies sold in over 30 languages. The game became hugely popular with the board game crowd in the U.S. Since then, tens of thousands of "new strategy" games have flooded the market. Blogs, websites, national conventions, "gaming cafes," where people go to play games from the cafe's massive board game library over a cup of coffee, or more often a can of Mountain Dew, with friends. It's become a huge thing and there are so many fun titles to play it's hard to know where to start.

    This isn't your mom's Monopoly or Clue game either. Settlers provides players myriad opportunities to strategically score points and win, by trading with other players and managing resources. Another of our favorites is Ticket to Ride, in which players collect colored cards to connect train pieces to historic depots along various country's rail systems, cutting one another off and scoring points for each connection. Karksonne has players drawing tiles to build the very board they play their pieces on to score points. High Noon Saloon pits cowboys and outlaws against one another in a saloon, complete with swinging fire pokers and broken barstools. In Tammany Hall, players don the role of 1930's mob bosses in gang-run New York City, vying for political votes from various racial factions, backstabbing, slandering, and buying favors from shady characters that show up throughout. We play together as Knights of the Round table against the encroaching forces of darkness in Shadows Over Camelot, completing legendary quests to combat the invading Saxons, the mysterious Black Knight, and find artifacts like the Sword of the Lake and the Holy Grail. Some of our Star Wars games can take up to six to eight hours to play, littering the table with mini-figures of ships, hundreds of upgrade cards, trajectory rulers, and other measuring devices. These usually involve a lot of math, and any one game may have hundreds of cards, scores of wooden tokens, coins, or many-sided dice.

    I'm boring you with all of this so you understand - playing these games while I was in the hospital kept me sane. It took me out of my environment into other worlds where I could focus on winning, conquering obstacles, working around problems, and finding alternate solutions to get ahead. The metaphor here is so obvious that I won't go into it.

And consider the games I played with the boys over Skype. Role-playing games (RPG's) like Dungeons & Dragons, Star Wars Age of Rebellion, and the like. Catharsis, escape fantasy, call it what you will. The fact that they warrant this much space in this story should highlight the crucial role they played in keeping our family engaged with each other, occupied, and me with something to look forward to during those bleak days.

It's Perry's first go at a modern strategy game, but he's a quick learner. He loses by a single point and he grumbles about it, then grumbles his thanks and thumps off to his room. Not to sleep. I awake at 4 a.m. to hear him clicking and sloshing around the circular hallway, and he doesn't wake until noon the next day. As I start paying closer attention, I notice him requesting various nurses at shift change, hanging out with the maintenance guys, and leaving the unit constantly - to the cafeteria, but more often the children's cafeteria, where the food is considerably better, and even up to the slushy machine on the cancer ward. It's like he owns the place.

Later in the week, I hear cursing and laughter coming from the open door to his room. He's ended up in the biggest room, across from the nursing office on the unit. The HVIC at Hershey is split into two wings. At the very rear exit of the hospital, you can turn right or left and enter one or the other of those. They are mirror images of one another. Rooms set along the perimeter of the oval shaped hall, with a massive open area in the center for desks, supplies, and the Pixis room where the drugs are kept. Needless to say, it's very noisy for patients, even with their glass doors slid shut - the beeping, the call bells, the talking at all hours of the night. The only exception to this mirror image is Perry's room. The right wing of the unit is shaped more like a giant "Q" than an "0," and the reason is because of room 1170. When the wings were converted to use as an HVIC, apparently there was a little extra room at the end of the outer hall on the right, so room 1170 is disproportionately large compared to the others. The next closest room has a giant window overlooking a gazebo area. This is Jamie's room. She's a small, red-headed woman who looks twice her age. She's reputedly destroyed her heart with narcotics, and we're acquaintances from my walks past her room over the last few months. 1170's large window only looks out to a brick wall, but it more than makes up for the crappy view with its size. It had been my room once, early on, but on that day, I realize that I'd not fully taken advantage of its size.

When I reach the door, I'm transported back to college. The massive hospital bed and boom that holds the supplies and computer are pushed flat against the wall, opening up the entire floor space of the room. This is occupied by Perry's chair, which has been turned to face the giant monitor, intended for X-Rays. Various chairs are gathered around the center of the room, occupied by Adam and Mike, and the screen is occupied by Madden 20-whatever. His XBox is connected to the monitor - or is it the PS3 or Wii? The room is littered with clothes, a mini basketball hoop hangs in the window, and the table next to the chair holds more condiments than you can find at a grocery store. Hot sauces especially. My presence goes unnoticed in the whooping and hollering. Perry, cursing the loudest, waves me to come in.

There is a rack shelf near the sink, piled with all manner of cooking pans, pots, and utensils. The supply cabinet above, doors standing wide, reveals not masks, gloves, or medical paraphernalia, but is crammed full of canned food, rice packets, soups, candy, soda cans, and boxes of breakfast foods. Dirty clothes, empty take out boxes, and soda cans litter every flat surface. The kid has literally moved in.

I don't stay long, but immediately start making plans for my next visit.

It's easy, that early in the relationship. We don't really know each other yet, and we talk about things you normally don't with strangers, using the shorthand that terminally ill patients share. We're all on fluid restrictions, interact with the same staff every day. We talk about our odds, the people we've already lost along the way. Relationships strained, and things we've had to let go of. He's nineteen, but he's been sick for ten years, and easily speaks of death, the toll his condition has taken on his family, his parent's marriage, his life experience. He's spent several birthdays and his graduation in the hospital. I have too - and anniversaries, kid's birthdays, and other occasions that should recall better memories than swans caths, blood draws, and constipation from the sedation. We talk a lot about needles, which nurses can be trusted with secrets, which doctors to appeal to for what. We rage against UNOS and HCM and the universe in general.

His mom and sisters live nearly two hours away, and his mom, Victoria, works all the time to support the family, Perry's dad having bailed out early on, when Perry and his younger sister, Samantha had a defibrillator placed at a young age. Perry rages against him too, and I learn that he's had to be the glue in the family, the one who helps the girls with their homework, parents them when Victoria can't, and deals with all the other cards that fate has dealt them. He shrugs off my awe as if it's normal for a teenager dying from HCM to do all of this.

"What do you cook with all of that?" I ask him one night in the middle of a Dominion match (a bloodbath, for my part).

"I made spaghetti for everybody last night," he says. "You didn't get any? It was in the break room."

"How would I have gotten in the break room?"

"You just open the door and walk in. I keep stuff in the freezer down there too. Nobody uses it." I've been coming here for about two years at this point and he makes me look like a newbie.

"You made it in the microwave?" I'm fascinated. Cooking your own food to avoid the slop in this place? Sign me up.

"Yeah - nurses chipped in to get me a bunch of microwave cookware. I make pasta all the time in there."

"How do you get groceries?" I ask, mystified.

"Joanna, Lori, some of the other nurses. I text them a list. They take my laundry home too." This revelation sparks an explosion in my head. What does a patient do in this situation about laundry? Bills? Haircuts? I know that Ryan cuts Perry's hair because he's good at it, but what if Ryan isn't here? What does Jamie do? Maybe that's why her orange hair looks like a shrub on fire all the time.

"I'm making BBQ Lasagna tonight if you want some," he says.

"That sounds disgusting, but yeah. And I want to help!" I blurt.

"Sure. Meet me about six."

And so I do. It's one of the best things I've ever eaten.

"Going to be one of the main dishes for my food truck," he says, mouth full.

He shows me pictures of the refurbished food truck his grandfather bought him for his last birthday.

"So, this is the dream?" I ask. I'm shoveling down the BBQ Lasagna and thinking, it's money in the bank if he can cook like this in a microwave.

"This is the dream. Working on the menu already."

He takes me online and shows me his tentative food truck menu, his branding strategy, and explains the whole vibe of the business.

"No way I'm going to college. I think I can make more money like this."

Conversations from Room 1170

I nod my head in agreement, my mouth full. Christie keeps me supplied with good food from home when I'm in here - how, I have no idea, given her continuing work schedule and keeping up with the kids and visits. But the Lasagna is good enough to sell, no doubt.

The two weeks pass, and I return home, having spent nearly every night eating with Perry in his room, playing board games and binging Scrubs reruns until the wee hours. Nurses join when they can.

I spend a day or two recovering, but I can't enjoy being home much, thinking of him sitting up there by himself every night, his family so far away. I won't be back for another six weeks. Maybe he'll get the call by then.

The boys miss him to.

"Let's just go," Rich says. "Why can't we just go see him, like visitors?"

I'm slow. It hasn't occurred to me that I can visit my own HVI. I've been driving a bit more, on and off, so why not? We spend the next day making a ton of food - garlic chicken, enchiladas, pasta, stir-fry, and sandwiches, and pack them up, along with a dozen games and our card table.

"We're coming up to play tonight, want anything from Turkey Hill?" I ask him over text.

His four-word reply, "Mountain Dew Slurpie. Big."

If he's happy to see us, he doesn't show it, ever the curmudgeon. But he eats heartily, asks if there's garlic chicken in any of the meals we brought, and we jump into a game of Tiki Mountain, in which he tricks Brennan into losing, then gloats. He's a terrible loser, and an even worse winner. We don't play Catan anymore. There's no point. After he lost the first time, he went online, watched a ton of strategy guides, and now beats us before the game even gets off the ground well. And then he gloats.

The boys pig out on his stash of Jolly Ranchers and Atomic Warheads, and we all go home sick from sugar and caffeine.

This becomes a regular activity over the next six weeks. At least twice a week and a few Saturdays, either the four or five of us can be found around the card table in Perry's room, eating Christie's food, or something criminally spicy we made together on his hotplate that violated four different safety protocols. He loves my favorite meal - Chicken Kali-Mirsh (Goddess of the Black Death), an Indian dish that calls for four tablespoons of black pepper per serving. Then we engage in some three-hour game of High Noon Saloon or Candamere. If we're too busy to make it up there, Christie deposits food to the unit fridge for him on her way to work.

The next time I'm in, I bring ingredients to make meals and we cook most nights in his room, resume our ritual of playing games until 2 a.m while Netflix loops American Dad or Scrubs on the giant TV in the background. He's essentially force-feeding Jamie at this point. She needs a TAH as well, but she's too small and weak for one, and a pediatric sized unit isn't patented yet. If she won't come to the room, we take food and sit with her until she eats it. She won't eat anything healthy, so Perry has resorted to crap microwave pizzas and flatbreads, chicken nuggets, and such. She at least gets a little protein down. He acts like it's his responsibility to make her eat, and any suggestion to the contrary, from me, her, or the nurses, is met with patient, but persistent silence.

He's also blown away by the food we're bringing.

"I need to have take-away lunches for my truck, like the ones you make. Once I'm up and running, we need to negotiate something, so I can sell them."

"I can't sell food I make at home, dude. We have a dog. Health department will freak out."

"So you make it in the truck. Maybe I cut you into the business. You've run a floor business before. You can cook. And God knows we're both going to need the money."

I turn this over in my head a bit. "I was thinking of culinary school on the other side. Maybe this would work instead."

This leads to several long, late-night conversations with note-taking, researching food and permit laws in the state of Pennsylvania, back and forth's over the web tweaking ideas for menu items. By that time, maybe Rich is old enough to drive the truck. He can make some money too. We start throwing around ideas for a logo, something to show that we're both transplant recipients, maybe find a way to get the Med Center to invest or advertise. Ideas abound, some practical, some fantasy. But it's a plan, and it's something to talk about other than the fluid restrictions and the PICC line infections. I lay in bed at night trying to imagine a life on the other side of all this. Working for myself again, making food, sounds like a good one. I've fallen in love with gourmet cooking, particularly making it affordable and portable, and bringing food to the hospital and to Perry has made me fast and good at it. For a time, Christie and I had even started a short-lived meal making business to pick up some extra cash between my admissions. Short-lived because I gradually lost the stamina to make the orders on time. But it's given me confidence that I can make money with food.

***

In room 1170, Dominion becomes the game. A deck building marathon with hundreds of different card varieties, the goal to collect as much property as you can and rob your opponent of theirs by the end. Jamie can only stand about ten minutes of it before she retreats to her room to watch trash TV. One night after she leaves, I tell him I'm worried about her. He cuts his eyes at me over the top of his hand.

"We're not all getting out of here. You know that, right?"

We stopped talking about death and fate a long time ago. It was easy to talk about that stuff when he was just the kid down the hall and I was the guy whose wife made the killer garlic chicken. Other heart failure patients pass in and out of your life constantly. You mourn them and move on, because you don't know them very well. You're kind of scared to get to know them, because when the worst happens, you see yourself and your family in that scenario and it all gets too personal. We'd lost Dottie a few months earlier. She'd been waiting three years for a heart that never came. She drowned in her own interstitial fluid - flash pulmonary edema, while sitting on the couch at home. I suspect her phone was sitting next to her, waiting for a call that was not to be. Her and twenty-something other people that day. Hundreds were buried the same day with perfectly functioning organs that could have saved not just Dottie, but six other people. Jo waited too long and suffered the same fate post-transplant.

I don't know how to respond to this sudden, confrontational assertion. But the kid's right. We know the statistics. We know UNOS. We know the stories.

"Yep." I don't know what else to say.

"Thing is, I don't have HCM anymore," he continues, playing and drawing cards. "But you do. I'm collecting time, living here. But you're never gonna move up unless you move in."

"I don't have just reason to. Insurance won't pay for it."

"I'm just saying, we talk big about what we're going to do after, but chances are, we won't be around to do anything."

"So why even talk about it?" I'd lain in bed many nights wondering this, feeling like an idiot for even daring to talk about after. I reminded myself of people who talk about heaven - no way of knowing if it actually exists but using the idea as a balm against the harsh cruelties of this world. A band-aid, and a dangerous one at that. Get too entranced with what might be and lose sight of what is. For an HCM patient, hope must be tempered with reality. You lose focus otherwise.

"I figure it doesn't matter in the end," he says with a shrug.

I put down my cards. "What are you talking about, dude? Of course, it matters. You've got sisters, your mom. I've got a family. It matters, maybe not to us, but it matters to them."

"What do you think they're going to remember, after, if it ever happens?" He's casual, calm, and I'm getting worked up. He almost sounds suicidal.

"What do you mean? They're going to talk about how we beat this. How we held out and got to the other side. Cue the Rocky theme song." I don't think I believed in an "after" at this point, but my pastoral thing kicked in and I feel like I'm trying to talk this kid down from the ledge. This isn't his personality. Where is this coming from?"

"Nah," he says, playing and drawing again.

"Nah? Then what?" I've lost track of the game by now.

He finally puts his cards down and looks at me, really looks at me. Maybe for the first time since I've known him, he looks me right in the eyeballs. It's unsettling and makes me uncomfortable, like he's looking right down into me, seeing everything.

"You're scared," he says.

"Of course I'm scared. You're scared, Jamie's scared, Blake's scared, Sherri's scared. We're all scared!"

"I'm not saying I'm not. But you're scared you're not going to make it to the 'after' part. You need to be scared about what happens between now and then."

"What, that I'm going to get kicked off the list or something?"

"We both should be scared about what they'll remember." He leans toward me, something I've never known him to care enough in a conversation to do. "We won't be special just because we got a heart transplant. Think about it. People get heart transplants every day. Whoopie. Who cares?"

"The people around us --"

"I'm saying, think about what they'll remember. That you had a transplant? Or are they going to talk about this part? This part right here? Where we're sitting around in these rooms, wasting our days away, dreaming up plans about how we're going to conquer the world in some imaginary "after?""

"Yeah, but man, you gotta have those things to make it to the after. If you don't have something--"

"We've got something - we've got our families. That's not what I mean. Look, we can't beat this, right? I've already got a one-way ticket. No heart comes in time or this machine fouls up - and it's done that once already, which is what landed me here - and I'm done. Your heart's crap. How long you gonna last? You can't even stand up without going white as a zombie."

Perry Jenkins, eternal optimist.

"Nah. The heart transplant isn't what your boys will remember. Or Sam or Holly. They're going to remember this part. The only way to win is to go ahead and be scared, but stare it down, right in the face. Right now? Everyone keeps saying we're brave. We're not brave. We're both cowards and we know it."

"I hate it when people say that."

"Because you know we're imposters. The brave thing would have been just letting whatever happens happen. Instead, we're in here getting caths, banking time, trying to save ourselves with these crazy desperate measures. That's not bravery. That's being scared you're going to die. That's us."

So, I guess he can see all the way down into me. I've known this from the start. I wonder all the time if there's any dignity in going to these lengths just to stay alive. I doubt it. I know that what my family has endured in all of this isn't due to my courage. It's because of my fear.

"No one cares about heart transplants, you'll see. But they'll remember how we did this part, right here. We don't have any control over the transplant part. That's Soleimani and Fran. That's their test. Our test is right now. This. Right now."

He plays some concocted 12-chain card combo that he's cooked up over this entire unnerving conversation, grabs the last property and beats me like a dirty rug.

***

I'm in the room that will eventually become Jamie's for the next year - the one with the window overlooking the gazebo and playground. It's small, but there's lots of natural light, which usually distracts me from the agonizing fluid restriction and helps me make it through the two weeks.

Usually.

I don't know why this time. It's just one of many admissions - dragging on, never-ending. I've gotten used to the caths, the environment...Perry and I have a routine now. I know the nurses well enough to keep up with their engagements, their pregnancies, their kids, their own medical ailments, the ups and downs and politics of the HVI.

I'm starting to seriously consider not coming back. I don't know why. I'm lonely, more homesick than I've ever been. It's harder to say goodbye to Christie and the boys every time they leave, and instead of using the time to blast through mixing songs, writing, or catching up on my stupidly long list of backlogged video games, I just sit and stare out of the window a lot and wander down to the other picture window by the break room late at night after saying goodbye. It's happening - the attrition. It's sneaky, but I really notice it this time.

A knock at the door. "We're the skin assessment team, mind if we come in?"

An older woman looks like an admin or some such, with two younger women in scrubs. They have that deer in the headlight look that marks the new crop of residents that show up in July. I have no idea what the skin assessment team does, and I frown in confusion.

"We have to check for bed sores and skin irritation this month," she says cheerfully, stepping into the room. "It's really simple, we'll just check your elbows and knees, things like that. And I have some students with me."

Now I'm a bit like a deer in the headlights, as they begin manipulating my arms and legs, taking off my socks to check my feet. Then the older one asks me to lean forward, so they can check the small of my back.

As I comply, I feel her finger dive two knuckles deep into the crack of my butt. My eyes go wide as she calmly explains to her students, "So there's no moisture here, and you always want to check for that. It gets overlooked and it can become a very serious source of bacterial infection."

They take this in with head nods while I sit frozen in my seat, trying to wrap my brain around what's happening. I don't even remember them leaving the room. A few minutes later I gather my cords, unplug Dr. Doo-daa and wander into the hall.

Perry is hanging out with Lori at the nurse's desk between our rooms. I must look stricken because Perry takes a step toward me.

"You okay, man?"

My nurse, Lori, jumps up and starts toward me as well, so concerted must be my expression.

"How do you know . . ." I start, then rephrase, "I think it's possible...I mean, how do you know if…"

"Dude, what's wrong?" Perry asks.

"I think . . . maybe . . . how do you know if you've been sexually assaulted?"

He takes a quick step back and Lori freezes.

"Dude, you've either been sexually assaulted or you haven't. That's like, a black and white thing. You don't have to ask...what the hell happened?"

Lori sits back down, and I relay the story to them. I get to the butt part when Perry bursts out in hysterical laughter.

Lori's laughing so hard she can't talk. When she finally can, she says, "Well, we should tell someone."

"Who would I tell --" I begin, but she cups her hand to her mouth and yells down to the next nurse station to Big Mark.

"MARK! DAVID JUST GOT MOLESTED!" She doubles over in laughter again, nearly in tears.

"What's a skin assessment team?" asks Perry. "Never heard of it."

"BY WHO?" Mark yells back.

"SKIN ASSESSMENT TEAM!" Lori answers.

"Hey! HIPPA much?" I ask.

"Like you're going to sue me," Lori gasps between rolls of laughter.

"Wait," I say to Perry. "You've been here how long, and you've never heard of a skin assessment team?"

"We have one," Lori says trying to catch her breath, "but I don't think they're here today. They usually tell us at the morning meeting if they're on the unit. HEY MARK, IS SKIN ASSESSMENT EVEN HERE TODAY?"

"Hold on, hold on." I turn to Perry, a bit frantic. "You're right there in the next room - they didn't come over there?"

"Nope," he says with a grin.

"THEY'RE NOT HERE TODAY," Mark yells back.

Joanna's hearing this now and gets the whole story from Mark.

"Skin assessment isn't here today," she tells us all.

"Wait, so some random woman, maybe from off the street just brought two girls into my room and stuck her finger down my pants? They may not even work for the hospital?"

This sends Lori into hysterics.

"Dave," Perry says in all seriousness. "You should do something. I know it's hard being away from Christie, but you'll survive, man. You don't have to hire women to come to your room for kinky stuff."

I walk off shaking my head. No empathy from this bunch. They've settled down by the time I walk my few laps and get back to my chair.

Another knock at the door and Larry, the cleaning guy, sticks his head in.

"Skin assessment."

It becomes a running joke over the next year and a half.

Conversations from Room 1170

***

For four months I observe Perry, this unexpected Yoda, his ill-advised obsession with professional wrestling, his love of unspeakably spicy hot sauces (sometimes fiendishly injected into the nurse's food or mixed into their drinks), his devilish pranks, his rebellion against being the conventional patient, his determination to be compliant at all costs, and the walking. The endless walking. You can't be in the hospital with Perry and not walk the laps. Eight-eight steps around the unit. Ten laps at a time, then fifteen when you've worked up to it. Are you going to walk when you get home? You need to. Force feeding Jamie with peer pressure, manipulation, and bribes. Walking, walking, walking. Walking and talking, walking without talking, walking with headphones on. Bringing Jamie food from the caf, trying to sneak in some protein. Walking when the unit's crowded, walking when it's vacant. I've never walked so much in my life and it saps the energy from me. But my legs stay strong, and I don't atrophy, like so many do. And Jamie doesn't waste away to nothing. No excuses. Not to Perry. You walk or you're persona non-grata in his book. Blake, another TAH patient who's become a friend, is in for a few days and I follow them in the endless loops, both of them thump-thumping in polyrhythms. Perry tries to scare me with stories of people drowning on the inside because they let the fluid buildup. Keeping up with your fluid restriction? Jamie, you? I know you hate it, but you don't want to drown. Walk, walk the fluid off. Remember Dottie? We gotta walk.

I wonder if he does it because he needs to or because he knows we need to. Or if he's just restless, and walking is the only way he feels like he's actually going somewhere.

Chapter 10

Suspended

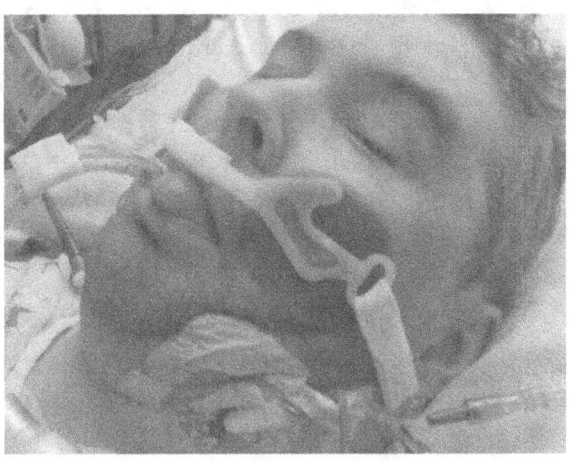

Suspended, I thought we were almost there
Life upended, one stop too soon, no time to spare
Suspended

Limbo, faith in a stranger's fate
A window, in a room of doors slammed in my face
I can't keep going, but I can't stay
One more gamble, the only way
Suspended, suspended

Can't move forward, I can't stay
One more gamble, the only way
One-way ticket, it's a fleeting hope
Fork in the middle of the only road

*Can't move forward, can't retreat
Huddled in the corner, skipping beats,*
Suspended

"You look like hell."

Dr. David Silber stands in the doorway of my hospital room, frowning at me. He's usually jovial, obviously Jewish - I always picture him wearing a skullcap, leading a Pesach meal, draped in a tallit shawl. Along with Dr. Popjes, Davis, Boehmer, and Clemens, he rounds out my cardiology team. I rarely see Silber, maybe in the clinic if I have to go there, but I normally see him in the hospital. It's been six months since I've seen him. We've developed a rapport over the last few years. Tall, gangly, a little physically awkward at times, goofy sense of humor.

"He's a socially awkward freak," Perry says dismissively. He's on the list of people Perry won't allow in his room (that list is chock full of social workers, therapists, phlebotomists, nurse managers, and even certain nurses).

I love Silber. He's spent plenty of afternoons with a chair pulled up to my recliner, talking about everything from The Hitchhiker's Guide to music to theology to string theory. He says I'm the most knowledgeable non-medical person he's ever met when it comes to HCM. My conversations with him over the years are largely responsible for that.

"No, really, Dave. You look terrible. I don't know if I would have recognized you. What do you weigh right now?"

"I was two-twenty-eight this morning." Fifteen pounds heavier than I was when I first came to Hershey. All fluid retention.

He quizzes me about my symptoms, my numbers, we catch up on our families and Disney buying the Star Wars franchise, and he takes his leave.

A few hours later, he's back with an older guy who looks like he just walked straight out of the operating room.

Long-term patients know when something's going down. It's a sixth-sense we develop over time, and the appearance of a new medical pro in your room or in the clinic is either a student or someone all the way on the other end of the spectrum. This guy isn't a student. As this registers, it also crosses my mind that this is a Tuesday, the day of the week when the entire cardiology team, docs, coordinators, nurse managers, surgeons, device techs, and intensivists meet to discuss each patient individually. Either a heart has come for me (unlikely) or something is very wrong. Am I getting booted off the list again? Silber's earlier inquiries about my symptoms suddenly feel like more than a friendly chat.

"This is Dr. Soleimani, he's one of our transplant surgeons."

So, something very bad. If I was getting a heart, the surgeon would either be at the recovery site inspecting the organ, or already in the OR, prepping for the procedure. And Silber's cautious tone tells me something's about to twist away from me again. I can see it in his body language and his demeanor is serious. Christie comes in before Silber says anything else. She gives me a puzzled look.

"We talked about you at our meeting this afternoon. I'm looking at your lab work from last Tuesday when we did the cath. Your liver numbers are really scaring me, and I'm concerned about your kidneys as well."

"Is it the meds?" I ask. Some of the stuff I've been on, particularly the Amiodarone to control A-fib is notoriously destructive to kidneys. That's what this is. I'm in liver and kidney failure and they have to take me off the list. This is it - no way I'm going to get multiple organs. My heart's too far gone.

"The heart function you have left is great," he says, "but it's not enough to keep you alive long-term. Obviously, or you wouldn't be here. It's not perfusing your liver and kidneys and they're starting to fail. The problem is, we don't know how long before that happens, and when it does happen, it happens *fast*."

"So, what do we do now?" Christie asks. Same question we'd posed to Dr. Maron on that awful day back in 2010. We both expect the answer to be, "there's nothing we can do." The fear of this whole journey ending badly has plagued us from the outset and looms every time we come to some new crossroad. I've been turned away so many times, it's like we're wired for rejection now. Wired for Rejection. Great band name, if I ever play in a band again.

"So, you've met Perry, I take it," Silber says. Everyone knows I've met Perry. We're like Abbott and Costello around the place, even when I'm not admitted. We've adopted one another's pranks and schedules. When the unit is crowded and we're doing our laps, we shout out "dead men walking!" to rattle the students and baby doctors.

I'm sure there have been Meetings and Discussions about us.

"You want to implant a TAH," I guess. I've been thinking about it for a while. Perry needs five hours of sleep a night, eats what he wants, and has little to no fluid restriction. He's walking around the hospital at a pace I couldn't have matched five years ago. It seems like a sweet deal. Except I don't want it. Surgeries mean blood transfusions, lots of them. Transfusions mean antibodies, and the more antibodies, the more risk of antibody conflict. It's a big enough danger in a transplant to begin with. Why double the risk?

The stoic Dr. Soleimani finally speaks up. "We think it would improve your kidney and liver function and make you a better transplant candidate."

Christie is stunned. I'm skeptical. I ask a few other questions, not even sure what exactly to ask at all. Silber wants me to have the implant as soon as possible. The rest of the team agrees. Even the "surgery-as-a-final-option-and-maybe-not-even-then" Dr. Davis.

I refuse to commit until I see my kidney and liver numbers and research problems related to heart failure and my specific meds. I've heard horror stories about centers, most famously the NIH HCM program in the 1990's, implanting patients with all types of devices without good reason. I'm savvy about kidney failure; I've been playing chicken with it for years on beta blockers and anti-arrhythmia meds. I know the numbers, I know what they mean and why they mean it. When it comes to the liver, Christie and I are both in the weeds. And Rich's fourteenth birthday is coming up in two weeks. I'd rather his present not be dad on a morgue slab. At the same time, I trust Dr. Popjes, Dr. Davis, and Fran implicitly. Even though I suspect they would have floated this idea if a heart hadn't come soon, it's the first time the reality of a chest-splitting, organ-removing surgery really takes hold in my mind. Christie leaves some food and heads upstairs to start her shift. This is always how these things happen. Some major decision to be made and she can't take time off, call in, or be late because her manager's leniency, though generous, is wearing thin. We'll talk about it after her twelve-hour shift, early the next morning, when she needs to be racing home to bed before doing it again. It's normal for her to stay with me until ten or eleven, until the doctors do rounds, before she finally agrees to go home and sleep.

No sooner have Silber and Soleimani left than here he comes, stealthy as a garbage truck at 3 a.m. Ka-foosh, ka-foosh, KA-foosh, KA-Foosh, KA-FOOSH. Perry and his adopted big brother/nurse Shaun appear in the doorway.

"You gonna do it?" Perry asks.

"You guys suck at HIPPA," I say, going back to whatever song from Instead of Wither I was mixing at the time.

"Ask a lot of questions," Shaun says cryptically before pulling the door closed, leaving Perry and I alone. He pulls up a chair. Perry Jenkins, Harbinger of Doom. Ready to counsel me on my trip to the abyss. It's times like this, I imagine Terry Pratchett's loveable Death character from his Discworld novels. Standing quietly in the corner, thumbing through the latest issue of People magazine. His perfect skeleton grin fixed on us both. Waiting patiently.

"You're going to get it," Perry says. "Here's why. Your heart is crap. It's got to go. We all know this."

"How do I know my liver and kidneys can't hold out until I get the call?" I'm grasping for any reason not to do it, already. One surgery, a transplant. One and done. I mean, who's ever heard of replacing your heart with a plastic one and just going on with life? Perry's nineteen. No job, no wife, no commitments. For me, the TAH seems like a sidetrack. One more complication, one more risk that it wasn't going to work out. I'd done my fair share of risk taking, thanks.

"Dude, you're never going to get the call. We both know this too. HCM patients don't get called. They either get it while they're here, or they die. You go back home, you're at the bottom again. I'm a 1B at home, even with this," he says, tugging on the cannulas that disappear under his shirt into whatever macabre rigging keeps them attached to the internal heart. Every time I see him do it, my stomach turns.

He catches my grimace and stands up, pulling his shirt high so I can see it for the first time. I don't want to see it, but I stare in morbid fascination. The two tubes disappear under a bandage on the left side of his abdomen. It's about the size of my hand, and through the transparent windows on the dressing I can see where the cannulas are stitched into him. A crusty brown film - he calls it "synth-flesh" cakes the tubes at the insertion point for about an inch, and the insertion points themselves are clean, though there are a few small scabs in places. Further down, not covered by the dressing, are joints in the lines where they can be detached, should the external pump fail and need to be replaced, or in the event he'd need to be placed back on the larger pump.

My stomach churns again and a million questions buzz through my head like a swarm of hornets. What if the machine stops working? What if the batteries run out? What if I accidentally step on the lines, or someone pulls them? What about the noise? I can't finish recording this album with the thing thumping and clicking non-stop into the microphones.

Then again, Perry lives with these risks and fears every day. Every day since I've known him, he probably worries about all of this. And he's nineteen. The kid's never even driven a car.

"You're going to get it because what does it matter anyway? The heart's got to go. Get rid of it now, feel better for a while, get more 1A time. And give your family a break for Chrissakes. Because we both know, the other organs go, and you're even more dead than you already are."

"We don't know that. There's no way to really know th-- I just need to do the research, okay? I need to know for myself."

"Bullshit. You're scared. Just say you're scared and get on with it. You think Eric or Fran's going to let them do this to you if it's not the right thing? Davis? Fran would be throwing down in the hall out there right now if she thought they were trying to sell you a machine you don't need."

He's right, of course. He's a pro-wrestling fan, so not without his flaws. But I know he's right.

"How long do you expect Christie to keep doing this? Dragging the kids up here?"

"The kids want to be here."

"Bullshit again. They want to be playing soccer and paintball and doing things with you. So, don't get the TAH, let your liver go. What about what they want then? You guys need a break. Get the heart. Heal up, go home, have a little bit of normal life for a while."

"How normal is it really going to be on that?" I ask, nodding at the TAH. "What happens if the machine fails?" But I know. Right now, normal is sitting on the couch all day, regretting that I'm not out riding bikes or going to the pool with them, waiting for the next fit of A-Fib, while they try to take care of everything else, including me.

"It's less likely to fail than your crap heart," he says casually. "The alarms went off one time and Holly (his little sister) was the only one there. I just got everything lined up, held my breath, and made the switch."

"What if you'd passed out?" I nearly yell. "That's crazy!"

He shrugs. "We're already way past our due date, man. What else was I going to do?"

"I don't know...we've got to talk about it. I'm not doing anything unless we all agree. The boys are coming up tomorrow."

"They're going to tell you the same thing I am." And he knows them well enough to know that too.

"And I want to talk to Joanna and Lori. They won't tell me what I want to hear, and they know how this has gone so far." My two no-nonsense nurses that have been with me from the beginning. By then, some of the ones I'd started with, Natalie, Jenn, and a few others, had moved to the progressive heart failure unit. I see them all the time, but they're not directly involved with my care anymore. Joanna and Lori had both gone toe-to-toe with residents and doctors over my fluid and med management. They are fierce.

"Yeah, sure," he says. "But you know you've gotta do it. It's your only way out of this mess. You know what your chart looks like."

"Do you?" Probably. I wouldn't put it past him.

He shrugs and opens the door. "Maybe, maybe not. I just know. I've heard things."

"YOU SUCK AT HIPPA!" I shout as he clicks and sloshes his way back down the hall to agitate someone else.

***

It's one of those mild mid-July summer days in Pennsylvania and we're sitting in the gazebo outside of the HVI. The five of us - my nurse Gale has to be there since I'm technically "off the unit." Four of us have been jousting back and forth for half-an-hour about the pros and cons of the TAH, whether I'll stay in the hospital or not after that until I get transplanted. What if I didn't do it, or did do it, and live on the HVI, like Perry, only to end up spending my final days on a machine, away from Christie and the boys, only to die waiting? Gale doesn't say much, just interjects when she has a piece of information that we don't. I don't want to make a decision until I know more. Christie isn't sure, and Rich thinks getting the TAH is the best thing at this point. Brennan hasn't said anything yet, as usual. When everyone has said their piece, he finally speaks up.

"First," he says ticking off a finger, probably following the outline he's been building in his head, "your heart's going to burn out, either now or later, but it's going to eventually. It doesn't make sense to let it take your kidneys and liver with it. Second, people live for a few years on the TAH. You can get it, come home for a while, even though you'd still be low status…"

"The doctors may write to UNOS for an exception to have you listed at a higher status if you go home," Gale says. "They probably will."

"Don't hold your breath waiting for UNOS to do anything for my benefit," I tell her. "I'd be happy if they'd just take down the dartboard in the conference room with my face on it."

By this time, we're jaded and resigned enough about UNOS and their bias against HCM patients that we can actually chuckle about it. But only a little.

"So, you go home," Brennan continues, "whatever status. We know you're not going to get called at home."

"Perry says no, and Fran agrees," I say.

"That's that," says Rich.

"So, you go home, and we get a break for a little bit, maybe a few months," Brennan says. "Then maybe they let you come back in and stay here until a heart comes."

"Why not just live here," Rich asks. "I mean, it's not what any of us want to do, but if that's the fastest way for you to get a heart, and less time living on the TAH, you should probably just do it."

"What if things go bad, guys?" I ask. "What if I get it, stay here, and that's it? What if this is the last real decision I ever get to make? Maybe I get the TAH, but I should probably go home so we at least have some time together in case something else happens."

"So, save yourself from the kidney and liver failure and spend some time at home," Brennan pushes. "You feel better and can maybe do a little more than you can now, like Perry. We get that time together, then when you're ready, you come back."

Christie and I look at each other. Do they get it? Someone will have to be with me 24/7. Supervised at all times, even when I'm sleeping, someone has to be able to hear the alarms on the machine. Someone who can change the pump in an emergency situation has to be with me. It's supposed to be someone over eighteen, but we all know Perry went home on the TAH and had to change out the pump on his own when an alarm was squealing. It's unspeakably dangerous because if an alarm is sounding, the patient is likely to be on the verge of passing out, having an Incident, or something worse. Unplugging the cannulas to switch the pump stops the artificial heart in the chest. So, you're essentially stopping your own heart and trying to restart it. I didn't want to put such a life and death burden on anyone else.

But Brennan is ultimately right, and so is Perry. My heart has to go anyway. Am I going to let it take my kidneys and liver on its way out? The TAH buys me time, but it's a one-way ticket. Once I take that step, it's straight ahead, either to transplant or death.

"That's where you're headed anyway," says Rich. We're somber, but there are no tears. Gale is amazed that we're having this conversation with our kids. But we have to. If I get this thing and come home, they have to understand the consequences of that decision.

"We've been building up to all of this," I tell her. "The transplant has been the main consideration for just about everything we've done since Brennan was two."

"They speak the language!" she says, laughing. "They know more about UNOS than I do!"

Rich shrugs. All I can think is that I wish they didn't.

"So, we're agreed," I say. "As long as Silber's numbers check out, get the TAH, come home if I can, reassess in a few months."

We agree it's the best plan we can come up with for now. These are the conversations I imagined that night in Virginia, sitting in the Italian place four years ago, when we'd first driven outside the reach of friends and families, on our way to Pennsylvania for Christie's first nursing contract. We've had others like this, about cardioversions, length of hospital stays, how to deal with all the little things that have popped up along the way. It's all led up to this. It's not like we were going to need to discuss the transplant when the time came. We were all on board with that, or we wouldn't have done all of this so far. If it hadn't been for all the other crossroads, decisions about where to take contracts, how to navigate procedures, responsibilities, and all the rest, the boys would have had no context for a conversation like this.

"But we're waiting until after Rich's birthday party," Christie reminds us.

"And I need to have a long talk with Perry. And I want to talk to Lisa (at the HCMA), Joanna, and Lori."

***

Rich's birthday comes and goes, and we do it right. A full-blown murder mystery with our friend Ron as a mad scientist, Jenn as a pulp-fiction detective ala N.C.I.S.'s Gibbs, and Marc Gecker as the mustache twisting cake poisoner that kills the caterer. The house is full of clues and kids, laughter, games, and friends. Much like Brennan's Psychonauts themed party back in March. It's a year for elaborate birthday parties. Who knows how many more we'll have? Maybe this was the last. It felt like it.

Christie and I get a bed and breakfast the following weekend and spend some time just the two of us. The meal makes me sick, like most meals do now, and I can't sleep at all that night with the nausea and shortness of breath. I'm glad we're together, but if it's the last time we have to ourselves I hate that I've spent it sick and miserable.

I quiz Perry and inspect every inch of the equipment, him giving detailed explanations of how everything works, what to be careful of (sitting to use the toilet - the zip ties that secure the cannula connections are sharp as razors), how to sleep, and everything else he can think of.

"Told ya you were going to get it," he says as I pop the spare batteries in and out of the charger.

"Shut-up."

Lori and Joanna don't think I need the TAH yet, but ultimately agree with Brennan's argument as I present it.

"You're saying you don't feel as bad as you are probably going to, and you don't look any worse, but I've been seeing you every few weeks for the last two years. And you have HCM. Why the hell are we even discussing how you look or feel? It's irrelevant. You'd better look at the numbers. BUN and Creatinine trends don't lie."

This is why I love Lori. Go with what you see, not what you feel.

"In a dark place we find ourselves," Yoda tells Obi-Wan Kenobi, hours after the Jedi Purge begins, *"and a little more knowledge lights our way."*

"Why are you asking me anyway?" Lori laughs.

"Brennan's smarter than all of us put together. And if Rich says he can handle things at home, you know he can. Is there anything you guys can't do? Look at what you've come through so far."

We have done the impossible, and that makes us mighty.

***

Three weeks before the procedure, my phone rings at 7 a.m. Normal for some people, but we're homeschooling, night shift people. 8 a.m. is like 5 a.m. to everyone else. I don't even have to look at the phone. Unless there's been some horrible accident in my family, it's got to be Perry.

"We're on," he says. "Surgery at 2 p.m." He actually sounds happy instead of grumbly for once.

"On our way," I tell him. That's it.

We're ready to leave in about twenty minutes and race to the hospital, hoping we'll be allowed in the room. It'll be like a tornado in there, I'm sure, but we want to see him before surgery. His mom and sisters came down earlier in the morning, but he'd waited as long as he could to call us.

The HVI is a beehive, and a happy one. Brenda, Lauren, Kim, Jenn, Mark, Shaun...how many people can say, "DID YOU HEAR?" before we even make it to Perry's room. Even Larry, my cleaning buddy is whistling as he flips a recently vacated room across the hall. Jamie is beaming as we pass her room. I stop to say something, and she waves me off.

"You better hurry. Soleimani's already come and gone."

The room is dark, no Family Guy or Scrubs blaring from the giant TV. His mom and sisters, Sam, Holly, and Rosie are lounging on the chair and bed. Holly, his youngest, is curled up in the bed with him. They've shaved his beard already and he doesn't look like himself, especially because he's grinning. We meet his family and it seems odd that we haven't already. They all run out to get some breakfast.

It's fast. The boys and Christie give him a hug. We do our fist bump, and I tell him I love him.

"You too, brother," he says.

I'm headed out the door and he says, "Oh yeah. I forgot - before you go in, they're going to shave everything."

"Yeah, I assumed." He looks five years younger without the beard. "See ya on the other side."

"Dave," he says urgently, leaning toward me from the bed. He lowers his voice, raises his eyebrows and nods down toward his waist. "I mean, *everything*."

I laugh out loud.

Perry's situation is different from ours. We're a half hour from the hospital and I see Christie all the time while I'm there because of her work shifts. Not that it isn't hard. But his parents are divorced, and I've never met his dad. I've passed his mom and sisters in the halls once or twice, but Perry doesn't share time with anyone else while they're there. They stay as long as they can during those times, all three of them sleeping piled up on the hospital bed while Perry sleeps in the recliner. It's expensive and difficult for them to come. They don't know us in the waiting room, so we introduce ourselves. They're quiet and worried. Perry's dad shows up, nervous and full of questions. We try to answer as best we can, but it soon becomes painfully clear that the family doesn't understand much about the transplant surgery, or how things are going to go down; but it's not their fault; most people don't. Between me being sick for a decade and a half and Christie being a nurse, we've had to know more than the average patient and we forget that most other people have been fortunate enough to have good doctors the whole time.

We're starving so we go grab food, then hit Wal-Mart and hastily throw together a basket of stuff for them to survive in the waiting room for a few days - toiletries, protein snacks, water, earplugs, and such. Christie, ever the nurse, includes digestive and other medical aids, and the boys pick out some things to keep little Holly busy. We drop the boys off and head back to the hospital. It's only been five hours, and with the TAH extraction, the surgery is more likely to take closer to ten. Perry's dad has left and returned, but he's acting funny and the family is ignoring his frantic pacing.

The hours tick by. Karen and Jenn swing through to update the family. I've known them both for a few years, but they don't acknowledge my presence. My gut sinks.

"The heart is in, but he's having some problems with the transfusions. Dr. Soleimani is staying with him and dealing with it, but it's going to be a bit longer. We'll keep you updated."

It's been nearly twelve hours at this point. I don't betray my distress to the family, but Christie and I exchange a worried glance. We're also ready to pull our hair out because the family doesn't ask a single question. We're notorious for asking too many, but we have no right to ask in this situation. I wish I'd gotten Perry's permission for direct updates.

Another two hours pass. It's nearly three in the morning when Dr. Soleimani comes in, haggard, terse.

"We've got him in a room. His liver and kidneys are struggling very hard right now, but the new heart seems healthy. I'm going to say with him because he also has a lot of fluid on his lungs and we need to get that off. But he is very, very sick."

Again, no questions. I'm digging my fingers into the seat cushion to keep from blurting them out. The minute the surgeon leaves the waiting room, I burst through the back door and race toward the front desk at the HVI. Brenda and a few others look up from their conversation and I put both hands on the countertop.

"He's very sick?!" I burst out. "What the hell does that mean, sick?"

Not that anyone would have been able to tell me, but only then do I realize that there's a nurse manager I don't know in their midst. She stands up and asks me if I'm related.

"Well, no, but..." I trail off, realizing how stupid I must seem, knowing they can't tell me, demanding them to anyway. They may not have known anything.

"Mr. Johnson," the nurse manager says, "we can only release information..."

"Yeah, I know. Sorry," I say, waving her off. She knows my name. Weird. As I turn to go I catch Adam's eye. His face tells me everything I need to know.

I linger in the main hall for a moment, trying not to vomit. The double doors open, and Brenda comes out.

"Sorry," she says. "I told her who you were. Sorry she was so…"

"It's my fault," I say. "I didn't see her there, and I know I can't ask you guys anyway. I just know it's bad."

I look up and she's wiping tears away. "I have to go," she says. We hug, and she disappears back into the HVI.

When I get back to the waiting room, Karen is explaining to the family that Perry's going back into surgery, now. He's bleeding, and his liver is going into failure. Dr. Soleimani needs to figure out what's wrong.

I can't tell if his family understands the implications of this, how dangerous it is. Karen explains that he's also on ECMO, to keep him breathing since his body's trying to shut down.

Something about this strikes me as funny. Perry's body can't shut down. He's too stubborn to let it. I'm delirious at this point, trying to convince myself that this is his greatest prank yet. We have to get home to the boys, so we tell Victoria and Sam (Perry's' mom and sister) that we'll be back in the morning as soon as we can.

It's fitful sleep, at best. How was everything so bright and happy just yesterday morning? Not that anything is very bright and happy when you're dealing with the waiting list, but the dark cloud had at least opened to a small ray of light for a few minutes. Now we're racing back to the hospital, filled with dread. We're met with mixed reports. He's back in his room, but he's in liver failure. No, kidney failure. No, both. Perry's mom is exhausted and hasn't been able to keep up with the reports she's been given.

Conversations from Room 1170

We hug them and go onto the HVI to find out that Dr. Soleimani, now going on thirty hours without sleep, is still in Perry's room, working on him. Karen had to get sleep, but Jena, no surprise, hasn't left his side since surgery prep the previous morning. Let them try to kick her out. I wasn't there, but I know what the two of them had agreed on. He'd made her promise to stay with him, and Jena, despite all hospital protocol and her own well-being, had promised. She may be sleeping on the floor in his room, but I knew she wouldn't leave until he was out of the woods or the worst had happened. I know this because when I ask if Jenna's still here, everyone nods. When I ask where she is, they just stare at me with glassy eyes.

It's the quietest I've ever heard the HVI, as if the call lights and bells themselves are holding their breath. No one knows for sure what's happening, but it can't be good. We don't know his family well enough to ask for HIPPA clearance, so we leave again. I want to sit in the floor outside of his room, because I know Jenna's staying, and I feel like I should too. But the boys are at home, and I don't want to leave them alone for long. They're holding up like they always do, but no one says much for fear we'll start crying. Everything seems like a slow-moving dream.

Weeks go by. We get bits and pieces, meaningful looks, overheard conversations, piecing together info from Sam, who's begun texting me on a daily basis. He's on dialysis, in an induced coma. There was a horrific antibody conflict with the transfusions, and his body tried to shut down during the surgery. The removal of the TAH had been bloody, though no one explained why until later. Loss of blood means transfusions. The more transfusions, the higher the risk of antibody conflicts.

With Perry in and out of stability and my own TAH surgery just a week away, it's hard to think about much else. The boys vacillate between introspective silence and obsessive video gaming. Worry and distraction. Rich and I talk about what will happen "if." We've just gotten settled in Pennsylvania. Will

Christie and the boy's move back to Arkansas? Will they have to go into public school? I don't know how to have this conversation with him.

Finally, we get word that Perry's been woken up. He's breathing on his own, but he's on kidney dialysis, very weak, and not surprisingly, very grumpy.

I make a quick trip to the HVI to see him, hoping he'll let me. I've heard that he's only letting his family, and Jenna and Krista in the room, Sam sometimes (all nurses). But they've got him and several other patients outside in the ambulance bay to get some sun. Carylon takes me outside.

I've been around sick people a lot. As a pastor, I've stood at the bedside of many dying people, some younger than me, held their hand, prayed with them. I've seen advanced stages of cancer and AIDS, liver failure, and horrible injuries from motorcycle crashes and drug-related beatings.

I couldn't have been prepared for what awaits me in the ambulance bay that day. Thin, yellow, eyes staring at nothing, he sits reclined in a rolling chair. I kneel down beside him and lay my hand on his arm, which he acknowledges with little more than a glance. He isn't able to turn his head to look at me, so I position myself in front of him, which means squatting on the hot asphalt to see his face.

"I'll be here in about a week, buddy," I tell him, then realize I sound like I'm talking to a child.

"Buddy?" Really, Dave?

He doesn't even roll his eyes at me, which bothers me more than anything else. He just stares straight ahead like I'm not there. "I'm bringing my Wire DVD's because I'm sick of making references you don't get, and we've got to catch up on American Dad. You've got to learn to play X-Wing too, Rich is dying to stomp you." Still no response. "Well, I'll come hang out once I'm in. I've got to spend a day or two before the TAH surgery…" I'm terrible at carrying conversations, and knowing Perry, he probably just wants to be left alone.

Carolyn uses her badge to let me back into the HVI doors and asks me if I'm alright.

"It's like he's not even in there," I say, my voice shaking.

"He is, Dave. It just hurts him to talk or move much. It'll get better."

"I don't think he even knew it was me."

She squeezes my shoulder. "He did. He's asked about you - he wanted to know when your TAH surgery was."

"Okay," I whisper uncertainly.

We part ways and I rush to the bathroom and lock myself in a stall and cry as quietly as possible for a few minutes. The boys are going to see him like this. What are we supposed to tell them now? This hulk of a person, who looms so large in our lives and minds, reduced to an unresponsive skeleton of himself. There's no way to shield them from it, not with me coming in the next week for surgery. They've known since they were old enough to understand that they're at risk for HCM. And I know they see themselves in Perry's place, in mine, and they wonder. How long before they're diagnosed with this dreaded disease and we start discussing assist devices, myectomies, ablations? Hopefully never, but a picture is worth a thousand words. And this picture is horrifying.

As for me, this was all supposed to end in a heart transplant, one and done, and we'd have resolution, one way or the other. This…this is a way station, an unexpected pit-stop along the way that we didn't even know to think about. We'd never heard of a TAH six months ago. Entering a state of limbo, suspension, where there is no resolution, only a one-way ticket to on a train that may run out of track before reaching its destination.

We've tried so hard to maintain as normal a life as possible for the boys in the midst of all of this, but it's impossible from this point forward to even pretend that things are normal. We have some idea of what this will be like from spending so much time with Perry.

The boys have held up under all of this with a resiliency that gives us strength at the darkest times. By my count, they've been left sitting in waiting rooms around one hundred times now, either during appointments or procedures, at least a third of those being risky. We're far away from the comfort of grandparents, and our friends all homeschool, so there has been no one to sit with them for distraction or support during those waits. Christie has been in and out, but they've spent the bulk of those times alone, with only each other for solace. At least a dozen times we've left them with friends in a race to the ER, them not knowing if I was alive or dead for hours at a time. Neither of them has flinched.

But Perry's complications, coma, and near catatonic state has pulled the rug out from under us all. In retrospect, it was a stupid and dangerous thing to do, but Christie and I, as well as the hospital staff, have held Perry up as a shining beacon of hope. He's lived on the TAH and gone on to heart transplant. If Perry can do it, the reasoning goes, so can I. But even that taste of hope has turned sour in our stomachs.

After laying in an induced coma for weeks, tubes in his mouth and nose, a machine breathing for him, he's finally awake. But he can't speak, can't walk… he's a shell of himself. He barely lets anyone in to see him, but he agrees to see the boys briefly before my surgery. He's bitter, angry, but mostly, he seems defeated. Who can blame him at this point? My short, one-sided conversation with him in the ambulance bay instills a dread in me - not for my own surgery, but for the boys. They know the risks, they understand the potential complications. They know that even under the best circumstances things can go horribly wrong. But that was all hypothetical. Now it's real. The fear made flesh. There's no use telling them I'll be fine, because they learned a long time ago that everything doesn't always go that way. They're not stupid.

We're embroiled in all of this the week before I undergo the TAH implant, and there's no protecting the boys from any of it. We've not been able to protect them from the gruesome parts of any of this, so we've compensated by going out of our way to protect them from unnecessary nonsense and pointless drama when we can, whether with the homeschool group of late, between Christie and I, or with family. I want to think it lightens the load just a little bit. They're still suffering the effects of the lapsed relationship with the Folsons, who've taken to passive aggressive barbs and jabs over the last few months. We're all confused and in pain, especially Rich, who's held on longest and tolerated a lot of ridicule and manipulation as a result. It's begun to affect our relationships with other friends in the homeschool group too. Perry has even been a solace from that, but now they feel cut off from him as well. They take it on the chin, but I hate it for them. Thankfully, the Geckers and the McCurdy's remain steadfast, as do several other families who've gone through the same cycle of intense friendship and subsequent rejection and slander by the Folsons. It's not our first time dealing with people like them, but it's the worst possible timing.

My parents decide to come for the surgery, while Christie and I tie up loose ends. We double-check my DNR (Do Not Resuscitate) order to make sure it's up to date. We've discussed this for years - no life-support for me unless the outcome is sure. I call Richard, my friend who pastors the Calvary Chapel where I used to serve, and we walk through a memorial service, chock full of U2 and Rich Mullins songs, and plenty of Douglas Adams and Terry Pratchett quotes. What little financial business we have is put in order, and I make sure Christie can access all of our credit cards, online pictures and such. In the days before the surgery, I finish recording a series of videos I've been making for the boys since the incessant A-Fib attacks in New Hampshire in 2012. I've set aside a jump drive for each of them filled with albums, my books, book and movie lists, pictures, and about a dozen videos from me with all the lectures and thoughts I may not be around to give; everything from girlfriends, to religion, to extended warranties. Along with a journal I've kept for each of them since the week they were born, this is what I have to leave them. I hope it's enough. There's a video for Christie as well that I hope she'll never have to watch. It's strange and difficult to think of what to say to someone from beyond the grave, but even the most awkward things are better than nothing. Or so I suppose. The most time-consuming task is finishing the mix and master of Instead of Wither at a friend's studio in Reading, forty-five minutes away. I don't know if I'll be able to do it after, or at all. Most people would have left the project unfinished but being that it's a concept album about my spiritual struggles over the last ten years, I felt it was imperative to at least get it to the point of listenability, even if it's never packaged properly.

It's been a mad race to get Rich's birthday done, have some time with Christie, and put everything in order before the surgery. We've had very little time as a family to just sit and talk about the surgery, what may happen after, what may happen if the worst happens. I can tell the boys especially need to talk about it. It's a bit awkward with my parents visiting, but the four of us take an evening to eat at Rodizio's (our favorite Brazilian place), just to have some final moments to ourselves before the craziness begins. We reminisce about the journey thus far, and I recall a similar meal, three years earlier, in a small Italian place somewhere in Virginia, when we were headed for Hershey. It feels like a lifetime ago. Where that meal was filled with excitement and hope, this one was filled more with dread, despite our best efforts to reassure ourselves that it would be fine. Our confidence is tempered by the image of Perry, sick and weak, burned into our brains. We talk a lot about life and death, my hopes for them should the worst happen, and what will come next if everything goes well. There are so many decisions to make in that case, and it does us all good to have our little family meeting and get it all out in the open. I drive home feeling like everything is in order, no matter what happens.

***

Perry was right. They shave *everything*. It's the morning of, and I lay sprawled on the bed in my room, razor buzzing, while an adorable little Puerto Rican woman tells me that everything was fine because "Chesus" has a plan for us all. I decide not to remind her that Chesus' plan for Isaiah was to be crammed into a hollow tree and sawn in half, or that his plan for Bartholomew was to be skinned alive while his wife and children watched. No matter anyone's theological stance on the Judeo-Christian God or Jesus, there's no disputing that God doesn't usually get very worked up over casualties when it comes to his grand plan, or that his plan doesn't revolve around us, contrary to Western thinking. So many theological fallacies to correct, so little time.

Christie, the boys, and my parents take turns listening to my heart one last time. Mudge and Terri drop by to wish me well and end up sitting in the waiting room the whole time, as does Brian. I don't remember much of that morning, other than wanting to get on with it. The main thing I remember when I come out of surgery is thinking, "No matter what, HCM didn't get me. HA!" My blog entries in the days following are more immediate than anything I can recall now:

Cyborg Dave, reporting in from Penn State at Hershey, PA. I've had a lot of very strange experiences in my life, but they all pale in comparison to this.

So, the first two days after admission, the docs tinkered with my blood, ran dozens of tests, and prepped me for surgery. When the day finally came there was lots of poking, prodding, and after a tearful and hopeful "see ya in a minute" to Christie, the boys, and my parents, I was off to the OR.

First things first - if someone ever says to you, "we're going to insert an A-line," do absolutely anything you must to escape. I didn't know what an A-line was and the experience will haunt me for the rest of my life. You know that soft, pale, innocent spot on the underside of your wrist that wasn't hurting anyone? Turns out, there's a huge artery below the surface that can be used to quickly administer meds, blood, etc. in emergent situations. And the ink pen sized needle used to access it must be inserted while you're awake. At about an 80-degree angle for some reason. I should have known something was wrong when they started strapping my left hand to a board and giving me small shots of local anesthetic. The anesthesiologist, Dr. Pasad, actually looked me in the eye and said, "I'm giving you lidocaine to numb the pain. It's not going to help. I want you to prepare yourself; this is probably going to hurt more than anything you've ever felt."

The man did not lie.

The actual insertion only lasted a second, but all the pain in the universe was packed into it. I now understand how people can pass out from pain. Good thing they hit it the first time because if they'd tried it twice, I very likely would have called this whole thing off. My threshold for pain has grown relatively high in recent years, but this was maddening, blinding pain unlike anything I've ever experienced. I don't know what came out of my mouth when he stuck it in - I remember something about the Pope and Jesus' mother. My back arched off of the table and I screamed whatever it was at the top of my lungs. Thankfully it was over quickly. I apologized to all the Catholics in the room, which Pasad dismissed. "I've seen guys twice your size weep for their mothers when we put that in," he says.

That was honestly the worst part. The sedation was deep, no time passed, and I woke up to the familiar sound of the TAH (ka-woosh, ka-woosh, ka-woosh), which told me immediately that all was well. A few faces swam in and out of focus - Tommy, the nurse that's cheered me on for the last year or so, John "the Mudgeman" Mudge, a fellow HCMer until his transplant a year ago. Christie, my parents, a few more nurses. The first few hours were blurry as expected, and the intubation tube not as bad as I'd dreaded. As soon as I was moderately lucid I was able to focus hard on my breathing, so they would pull that thing out - which they did after a few hours. Then blessed sleep.

I really don't remember many details from the last few weeks - I was on narcotics for the first eight days, and being such a cheap date, they lingered in my system for about two weeks. It's only in the last few days that I've felt like myself mentally, able to think clearly, and have a conversation without babbling a lot.

Currently I'm tied to a large machine that houses the TAH. Since I've been stable on it for a few days now, it looks like I'll get my portable version in the backpack hooked up tomorrow. This has been a challenge because I'm used to being independent, even while in the hospital. I've had to page the nurses for everything from dropping something, to needing a drink, to going to the bathroom. Bed to chair - chair to bed. I walk around the unit a few times a day and enjoy being able to go outside with Perry and eat Freeze Pops in the sun. He's doing better too, though he has a long road ahead with lots of rehab. But we're getting each other through this.

With my backpack, I'll be able to walk around the hospital (accompanied by a nurse), to the caf, outside, and move around my room on my own. Blessed independence. In the meantime, Christie has been faithful as always to bring me good food, hard candy, entertainment, and keep my cooler stocked with sports drinks. I've spent a lot of time watching Beatles documentaries, The Wire, and cooking shows, reading Pratchett when I'm lucid, and napping.

We also start the education part of the TAH tomorrow. Family and a few friends have to go through five days of two-hour classes to learn all about batteries, alarms, changing drivers, changing cannulas, power conversion, and all things to do with making sure I do my part to keep the TAH working properly. I can't express how humbled I am that people will take *that much time out of their lives for this.*

Rich is more eager than anyone to learn it all. I don't understand the whole "be a parent, not a friend" thing people have with their kids - I can't help but be this guy's friend, because he treats me like one. He's faithful to me not just because he's my kid, but because we genuinely like each other. I'm so glad our relationship has developed in this direction because I literally couldn't have survived the last two years without him voluntarily taking on a role as secondary caregiver (behind Christie) in my daily life. I love my son, but I also love "that guy" in a whole different way that makes me proud to call him my friend. Anyone should be so lucky to have such a friend. I could say the same thing about Brennan.

I can't say much about Christie here without getting really sappy. I feel like we've fought this war together, in the privacy of our own lives, and the experiences are too personal to share. Besides, I want to keep them - we earned them, and we will lock them away along with all the things that have turned our friendship into a happy marriage over many years. I would like to say that I would have been so faithful and tireless in her position, but I fear I wouldn't - I don't think I'm that strong. I doubt anyone is.

***

Stress runs high at home during all of this, ending in an uncommon conflict between my parents and Rich. It seems resolved, but the timing is terrible for everyone. I do the best I can to help work through it in my drug-induced state, but it leaves everyone incredibly frustrated, especially the nurses, who worry about my stress level in the days after surgery. I get to know one of the new nurses, Jerrod, very well, when I poop myself after a few days of laxatives. He's used to it, I'm mortified, and we agree that when this happens again, he'll be the one to help me with it.

I've left the nurses alone as much as possible for the past few years, being self-sufficient when I can. Since I've always been mobile after swans caths, I even change my own bedsheets and walk around to find them when I need something instead of bugging them with a call bell.

"You should just hit the bell - we're here to help with this stuff," Krista tells me on a regular basis.

"Oh, don't worry," I assure her, and everyone else. "The time will come when I'll be the one hitting the bell every five minutes, driving you crazy. I'm just storing up goodwill for when the time comes."

And I have. Everyone is really patient and I'm on my feet soon, Nate at my side in case I fall. Christie has a video of my first walk in the hall with him. I pause at Perry's doorway. He's propped up in the bed watching wrestling or some nonsense as usual.

"Let's get outta here!" I say.

He rewards me with a grin.

"Love ya, brother." I don't remember his response, but I move on and do a lap around the hall. It exhausts me, and I sleep the rest of the day.

Christie's parents come for a week or two, her mother cleans the house from top to bottom to prepare for my homecoming, and they head back for Arkansas. Mudge visits a lot, as do Marc and Ellen and Brian Ditzler. I see the boys about every other day, if not every day. Christie's working through most of this, not getting any sleep as usual.

Once the education is finished and we're given the green light, I finally get to go home. My first priority is eating some crab legs, so we call the place to make sure there's a table with a nearby outlet. No one ever understands why we're asking, but when they see me with my backpack, they get it.

I don't know how to feel. This machine has bought me possible years, saved me from multiple organ failure, and should bridge me to transplant. But how long will that be? Blake's been living with one for almost a year. Perry went for fifteen months. Can I do that? I don't have a choice. No going back now.

And it's a machine. As much as the bio-engineers, doctors, and techs assure me that these pumps are dependable, there are alarms and warning lights right there on the face of the thing to alert us if it fails. The training even involved the EMT company down the street from my house. But really. If the pump just shuts off without warning, how long do I have? Brain death after how many minutes? The pump can be replaced with a back-up, but between someone calling the EMT's and their arrival, eight, ten minutes have passed? And if the backup unit malfunctions, or the problem is actually with the heart mechanism itself, what is an EMT going to do? CPR? Epi-pen? None of that applies here; we're in uncharted territory. And despite the appearance of confidence from the staff and support team, it's obvious that everyone knows it.

This becomes painfully apparent the week I go home. My Aunt Vicky, who baby-sat me when I was three, is trained on the equipment and baby-sits me again while Christie's at work. She's here for a few weeks from Tennessee, but the TAH requires so much attention, I don't get to see her much. Three days after leaving the hospital, I return for an INR check - the machine is extremely sensitive to blood coagulation, so my blood has to be checked by a finger prick three times a week - and my number is low, landing me back in the hospital for blood and monitoring for another week. She visits me with the boys on the HVI, but I'm frustrated, expecting life to be more "normal" now that I'm stable and safe from A-fib and HCM. Once I'm back home again, I'm disabused of that notion within a day.

There are several things we have to stay on top of at all times. First, my INR number has to be in a certain range. It can be affected by leafy greens, or anything with a chocolate powder base

(Instant Breakfasts, protein shakes, etc.). Our lives become dictated by my INR number. We schedule around the checks, and don't plan anything because there are three chances every week for me to land in the hospital if the number isn't right. Secondly, I have a PICC line inserted into the underside of my right arm. This was done because I need blood draws every week until transplant, and my veins have become so trashed that even Dave, the hot-shot, one-stick wonder in the hospital lab can't hit me anymore. The PICC line runs right up to the edge of the TAH cavity in my chest, so the insertion site and surrounding area has to stay clean, dry, and occluded at all times. The site has to be cleaned and the bandage changed every week. Thirdly, the insertion site for the TAH cannulas are essentially open wounds, heavily bandaged, and the site has to be cleaned with a stinging chemical called Chlorhexidine. All of this takes up an enormous amount of time. I'm awake during the day. When Christie works she sleeps during the day. There's not much time between twelve hour shifts to fit all of this in, so we try to plan strategically around her schedule, but it changes often and there's no way to avoid conflicts.

We try a home health nurse at first, but it's too expensive, and it takes her an extremely long time just to draw blood and change the PICC line dressing. It takes a full day to get results back, which makes everyone nervous because of the INR issue. These nurses aren't particularly good, they aren't really TAH savvy, and it takes them far too long to enter everything on their laptops. I sit sometimes for two hours waiting for them to type, while my part only takes about half an hour. And they can't even change out the TAH dressing, which Christie and the boys have learned how to do. We give up on using home health after about a month, because of the expense if nothing else.

This means an hour-long round trip to the INR clinic three days a week, but the PICC dressing changes and blood draws are complicated. No one knows how to set any of this up at first, not even the coordinators, highlighting again that the Freedom Driver for the TAH is painfully new technology. In fact, we learn that I'm only the sixth person in the country (behind Perry and Blake) to leave the hospital with one. There is no standing protocol for blood draws or PICC dressing changes, and hospital red tape makes it impossible to do them through the obvious channels (labs, clinic, etc.). Christie finally strikes upon the idea to have the blood and dressing work done at the cancer infusion suite at the hospital, where cancer patients with similar issues are treated. We establish a routine; INR clinic Monday, then again Wednesday along with blood draw and PICC dressing change at the cancer center suite, INR again on Friday, followed by a quasi-shower and TAH dressing change at home. Believe it or not, the PICC line cleaning and dressing change in my arm is the most painful of all this. Luckily, we consistently end up with Jenn in the infusion suite. She's incredibly gentle and it makes that whole mess far less painful that it should be. As tired as we are, she's a bright spot in the middle of every week for us, always smiling and super-efficient. I still drop by the cancer suite to say hello, three years later.

All of this is further complicated by the fact that Christie has to drive me everywhere, since I'm not allowed behind the wheel. At least two of these days, she drives the half hour home after working for twelve on her feet, showers, takes me the half hour back to the INR clinic for a five-minute procedure, then back home to sleep before getting up to work another twelve. On Wednesdays when we add the PICC line and blood draw, we don't return home until after one o'clock, meaning she gets roughly three to four hours of sleep before going back to work another twelve. She's either working, driving, or sleeping, exhausted all the time. This goes on for four months. Friends offer to take me but are terrified to be alone with me away from home - which actually means they are afraid to be solely responsible for the TAH should something go wrong. It makes Rich nervous too, so he accompanies me anytime someone else does the driving.

Which brings me to the other challenge right now. I can never be alone. Not ever, not even for five minutes. If the Freedom

Driver fails, someone has to do an emergency replacement as fast as possible. This means the entire pump has to be changed, which means that between the time that the failing pump is disengaged and the new one is connected, the artificial heart totally stops beating. It stands to reason that I wouldn't and shouldn't attempt this myself (despite Perry's thrilling heroics. But he's Perry. I'm not.) because if the pump alarm is sounding and it's malfunctioning, there's a very high probability that I've already passed out. If I haven't, I could pass out in the moment between disconnecting and reconnecting the cannulas between pumps. This is a quick way to get dead.

So, I'm never alone. If I go to the bathroom, someone must be close enough to hear the alarms. Christie and the boys can't just run to the store - I have to go with, or someone has to stay. If I go to bed upstairs, the TV downstairs can't be so loud as to drown out my voice or the alarms, so someone usually has to come upstairs with me. We adjust to this fairly quickly at home, between the four of us. When Christie leaves for work, it's a whole different scenario.

Several friends are gracious enough to go through the training, so they can stay the night with me when she's at work. And we depend heavily on them to baby-sit me those nights. We'd bought a three-bedroom house specifically because we knew there would come a time like this, when someone may have to stay with me for a variety of reasons. The guest room is always occupied with people coming and going. We're incredibly grateful at first, and we still are, looking back. But between the constant TAH/Dave maintenance, and having house guests four nights a week, we're completely disconnected and stressed to the limit by November. We've been living for three months with constant company, like ships in the night. Christie and I are limited to talking during our drives to the hospital and back, when she's running on fumes. When she's off work, she's busy with all the responsibilities I can no longer keep. On the nights we have company, I just want to vegetate and watch TV, play a game, or nap. With one or two exceptions, our guests typically want to "hang out," - visit, go out to eat, chat, and watch movies. For them, it's a fun visit with a friend, and it's well-meaning. For me, it becomes another night when I need to be "on" and in

entertainment mode. That dynamic poses a threat to relationships.

Rich brings it up first.

"I think we'll be fine if no one's here," he says to me one day between school work.

I'm very reluctant to discuss this because though we've not voiced it, we all know that the boys are truly the ones "in charge" of the TAH should something go wrong. Despite everyone having been trained, they immediately start deferring to the boys anytime something happens, as they're the ones living with the lights and alarms and battery changes day in and day out. They also scored higher on the training final than anyone else after the medical personnel. In reality, the adults are only staying over as a buffer. Should the worst happen, I don't want the boys to feel responsible for it. I change the subject.

But another week passes and I'm growing more exhausted and temperamental. We all start to realize that our friends are becoming accustomed to the TAH, way too comfortable. Familiarity to the point of sleeping downstairs, not waking up to alarms, and losing sight of the urgency of the situation. We don't blame them. We're exhausted from the vigilance, but the boys are the most attentive of us all. They hear every alarm, they keep up with battery times and charging. They even pay attention to what I eat.

After a long discussion with Christie, I wait for the subject to come up again. It doesn't take long.

"Have you and mom talked about us staying home with you?" Rich asks again.

We're sitting on the couch, Rich, Brennan, and I. I don't get far into explaining why I don't want to.

"But we're the ones who are responsible anyway, Dad," says Brennan. "If something happens, anyone who's here is going to ask us what to do. And they'd probably rather us do it than them."

"And it's not like we're going to stand back and give them instructions," says Rich. "I'll feel worse if you die and I left it to someone else to change the pump. I'll always wonder if it would have gone different if we'd just done it."

"But I don't want that responsibility on you guys. You shouldn't have to bear that." I feel like a child, his parents trying to reason with him. Knowing I've already lost the argument.

"It doesn't matter how it should be," Brennan says. "This is the way it is."

"I'm not saying I like it," Rich says. "But Brennan's right. This is how it is, and wishing it wasn't won't change it. You and mom always say we have to deal with what's in front of us. And this is what's in front of us."

"We don't know how this will all turn out," says Brennan, "and if this is the last bit of time we have together at home, none of us want it to be like this. We want to be able to do the things we want to do, and not be stressed out and have guests almost every night."

It's a long silence. The implications of the two of them being responsible for the TAH - the TAH? - it would make them responsible for my very life. But they're right. They're already on the hook for that, like it or not. Adding other adults to the situation has only been a lame attempt to cloud the fact that it's this way.

"I never dreamed when all of this started, before either one of you were born, that I'd be here...and that you..." is all I get out before breaking down into sobs. They both hug me until I can calm down and talk again. It's the first time in all of this that I've broken down in front of them. Or maybe ever.

"It's not right," I manage to get out.

"None of its right," says Brennan. "It just is."

We explain the situation to everyone, but we decide to continue having Michelle and Dominique over a few nights a month when Christie works. They've become a fixture in our lives since we've moved here. We'd crossed paths with the Arnold family many times in our visits to Lebanon over the years. They're old friends of the McCurdy's and had been in our homeschool group for a while. The boys have gotten close to them both. We don't know they're here half the time; Michelle sits alone in the corner on her laptop while the kids play. My kind of anti-social evening.

The following weeks are comparative bliss. We eat in peace, watch movies, play games, have friends stay over a few times, but much less often. It's like old times. Kind of.

I think of when we started out from Arkansas, five years ago. On these nights when Christie worked, we occupied ourselves watching kid movies, playing hide and seek around the tiny apartments, the boys doing the appropriate "boody dance" when they were able to escape my searching. I always made smoothies and read to them before bed. They've outgrown the reading, and there are no more Lego marathons, or hide and seek for that matter. We play games still, but they're online with friends a lot in the evenings. I used to take care of them. Now they're changing my batteries, keeping me plugged in, bringing me things I need so I don't have to hassle with getting up and dealing with the TAH. I'm usually so exhausted that I drift off to sleep on the couch long before bedtime.

It could go on this way for years. Even with the TAH, I'm still second tier priority on the waiting list as long as I'm home.

Conversations from Room 1170

* * *

Perry's in the HVI getting dialysis for kidney issues. His sister, Sam has begun messaging me, but isn't quick to respond. We visit the HVI a few days into the New Year after one of my PICC dressing changes. He's covered head to toe in blankets while getting dialysis because it makes him cold. I try to lift up a corner so I can see his face.

"Don't," he says. "It lets the cold in." Grumpy, as usual. I don't realize at the time how bad he probably felt.

"Deal. But you need to answer your texts. Or call me. I don't know what's going on."

"Okay. I will."

Presumptuous of me to feel I have the right to know what's going on. The exchange is awkward, probably because I don't understand everything that's happening. The steroids, post-surgery depression, anxiety about the continuing dialysis, and who knows what else. But he seems cold and distant, and not in the usual Perry way. I don't know what it is, but it seems like something's changed.

He's readmitted the day after Christmas with pneumonia. Deadly for transplant patients - but it's Perry. He's been to rehab, gone home, and is getting back to normal life. HCM didn't kill him, so good luck pneumonia. You better bring your A-game. I dare anything to try and kill Perry Jenkins.

We go to see him, but Gail has to negotiate with the docs to get us in the room. They've put him back on ECHMO, to relieve the burden on his lungs, but they can't figure out what's going on. His head is raised, tubes running everywhere, in an induced coma. What I don't expect is the nurse from a team I don't recognize, running blood bags in and out of the room. They're giving him blood? I suddenly realize she's not only bringing blood bags in, she's carrying full bags out as well. Several times in the few minutes we stand at his bedside. How can he be losing that much blood? I pat his hand and realize there's blood under the nails too. I don't remember what I said to him. I couldn't grasp that he could be losing this much blood this quickly. I make it past the chapel and out to the sidewalk by the garage, and collapse into Christie, sobbing again. This doesn't seem possible. Perry's too stubborn to let this happen.

We don't say much about our visit to the boys other than that he's very sick. They're too busy baby-sitting me and taking care of the house and their schoolwork to think much of it at the time. He's been sick before - he'll bounce back like always, I convince myself.

For all the debate about whether or not I should live in the hospital following the surgery, it turns out to be a moot point. Sunday, January sixteenth, one day before my forty-sixth birthday, I get up early, as is my habit after adapting to hospital life. We've been in an ongoing painting project since we moved in. I've been in the hospital so much that it takes forever to finish any project. I pick up painting the trim in our sunroom where I've been working on and off. I've been at it a few hours when Brennan wanders downstairs. I'm cutting in an edge with purple, and when I turn to dip the brush, the world flips on its side. My stomach lurches and the room starts to spin. I drop onto a bench and start retching, violently.

Brennan comes running and immediately checks the TAH pump. No alarms, no lights; it looks perfectly happy. I'm positive that the device has malfunctioned, and this is how I'm going out. Not behind a drum set, or surrounded by my loved ones, but in the middle of painting the stupid sunroom trim, the project that taunts me with its perpetual un-finished-ness. Brennan wakes everyone up and Christie calls Fran, tries to get me up to go to the ER. But I can't even stand. I'm having full-blown vertigo and can't even tell where the floor is. Ten minutes pass and I'm still retching. All of the preparation, the training, the drills, confident we can handle any Freedom Driver emergencies, and this damn machine is going to kill me without making a single sound.

Chapter 11

Needlebeast

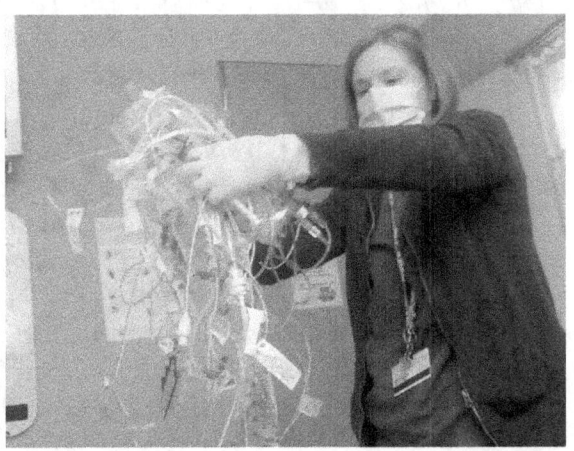

Here it comes, here it comes, zooming in again
Push hard, the tourniquet squeaking
Warm it up, hot packs and cold grins
Bull's eye or torn and bleeding

Dig deep, dig around, bruise bound,
Today we're Oh and Fifteen,
One will, one way, one road to pain,
White knuckle, blown and screaming

So many ways to drown a man,
So many ways to drag him down

Needlebeast, come and feast, (you can gorge on me)
Needlebeast, it's the least I will suffer

Conversations from Room 1170

Needlebeast, come and feast, (you can choke on me)
Voodoo doll, prick me – but I don't bleed

Come a tap tap tap tappin on the door
Last time around, we need a little more
Red carpet walk for all the Stick Stars
Can't catch me, I don't care who you are

Roll rider, ride the wire, skin and flesh through the fire
Blunt trauma, midnight drama, never come when they call ya
Small gauge, sideways, thread the scars, thread the maze
Dry well, tunnel blown, blood from a stone stone

(Hanging out here on the ropes, skeptics better learn my name
Shine and shimmer in the hope, laying face down in the pain
Eye on the prize, the do or die, never mine to question why
Means to an end, caught in the spin, blow it out and go again
Veins of steel, I've got the will, limping up another hill
Black and blue and red again, pick your poison, pick your sin
Bear the sting and ride the wave, treading in a sea of pain
Clench my teeth, face the day, it's the price we have to pay)

By the time the EMT's arrive, I've been dry heaving for a good fifteen minutes. Every time I open my eyes I start retching from the vertigo. Brennan and Rich are launching into the familiar routine of packing for a hospital trip; let the dogs out, grab phones, a few granola bars, my backup equipment, and most importantly, whatever Terry Pratchett book I'm reading from my bedside table.

It takes a second to sort out the riding arrangements. Christie wants to stay with me, but she can't be trapped at the hospital without a vehicle, plus, there's no way the boys are staying home for this – they probably understand the TAH and Freedom Driver almost better than Christie. Rich ends up in the ambulance with me and Christie follows in her car with Brennan. I'm nearly unconscious from the nausea and vertigo.

"We're going to give you some Phenergan through your PICC line," one of the guys tells me while unzipping the backpack, "Is that okay?"

"He can have that," Rich says. "But there are two ports; make sure you use the blue one. It's for meds. The other is for blood."

The EMT looks at the pump, then studies Rich for a second. Several people from his company were trained on the TAH before I was allowed to leave the hospital back in September, in case of a situation just like this. It's obvious from the look on his face that he has no idea what he's dealing with, but he nods and goes to work.

"Check. Blue's an entrance, red's exit," he says. "So if he goes into V-tach, what then?" Epi-pen?" This is a pointless discussion – it's not a real heart. It can't go into V-tach. It will just turn off.

"Won't do any good, probably the opposite." Rich squats down next to the EMT and starts pointing at the numbers on the read-out. "As long as the heart rate doesn't change too much here, the TAH is working. The fill volumes, here," he says, pointing again, "well…they measure the fill volume. They look right. That's why we're confused."

"Do you know what to do if the pump fails?" The EMT isn't sweating it. I'm sure he's seen worse. I just don't think he's ever seen something like Rich.

"Yeah, here." Rich says, unzipping the bag with the spare pump. He gives the guy a two-minute TAH 101 course.

"That's a lot to remember."

"It's not too complicated. I can walk you through it."

The nausea starts to pass, and I wonder if my fixation on the detail painting hadn't caused some kind of dizziness that my artificial heart couldn't adjust to. I sometimes get a little sick to my stomach when dealing with intricate details in Photoshop or Cakewalk (recording software). Maybe it has nothing to do with the heart.

I've grown to recognize what I call "TAH terror" among medical personnel. When I'm rolled into the ER, all eyes turn, filled with said TAH terror. They're all watching with rapt attention, praying to Jesus, Allah, Buddha, and any other god they can think of that I'm not going to end up in one of their rooms. None of them recognize the machine I'm attached to. They don't want to be responsible for it.

A groundless fear. Dr. Brehm, Dr. Pabst, Tina, – the device coordinator - and several residents appear within minutes with the big pump on wheels. I brace myself for the bizarre experience of the heart stopping for a few seconds as they transfer me from the portable Freedom Driver back to the rolling monster. It's the third time I've switched back and forth so I'm slowly getting used to it. I think Tina's more nervous than me.

X-rays. Driver interrogation by bio-engineering. Blood cultures. The blood's got to be a fresh draw - not from the PICC line. That means we need Dave from the lab, but of course, the ER nurses had to give it a go four or five times before giving in.

***

A word about needles.

My first serious experience with needles was in the fall of 1998 when I went for my very first heart cath in Little Rock, Arkansas at the Heart Hospital under the care of Dr. Van DeBryun, who I've previously mentioned. My prior experience with needles involved childhood vaccinations, some boosters when my dad was assigned by the U.S. Air Force to Northern Italy, and a painless

T.B. test at nineteen when I went to work for the U.S. Airbase youth center programs.

If you've ever had an IV placed, you know it's significantly different from getting a shot or having blood drawn. The shaft is plastic, and stays inside the arm, after the needle used to get it into the vein is removed. It's attached to a tiny tube and the whole thing is taped down to your arm, so you don't accidentally rip it out - because the other end is usually attached to a machine that's administering sedation, saline, or some medication.

It's much more painful than a normal needle, and is psychologically unnerving for me, because of the fact that it remained inside of me. I shudder now even writing the phrase "inside of me" (yes, me, the guy who's had over thirty swans caths left in his heart for two-weeks at a time and had a total artificial implant). The second time I had an IV put in, the nurse missed the vein, and the thought of it turned my stomach so badly, I almost blacked out. The team had to wait an hour before they could try again, and they called for their "best guy" (there's always a "best guy" - why don't they ever send him FIRST?) who stumbled into the room, Mr. Mago style and pretended to grope around as if he were half-blind. I was not amused.

Needles became a big problem for me when I arrived in Boston and began to be seriously evaluated for transplant. I needed blood draws at every visit. By the time we were living in Connecticut in the summer of 2012, I was having blood drawn every other week at the time. This trend came and went over the years, and I never got used to it. Every single time, I had to talk myself through it, look away when the needle went in, and focus on anything other than the fact that there was a foreign object inside of me.

When the needle came out, I fought the wave of nausea down and no one was the wiser. It was an internal crisis that I battled mightily for years. I wish I could say it got better with time, but it really hasn't. I just have to be sure to have something solid on my stomach, and some sugar on board, and I can muddle through.

There's an entire genre of horror film known as "body horror." Whereas classic thrillers scared audiences with the beast without - Dracula, Freddie, birds, and what have you, Body Horror films terrified audiences by placing the threat inside the body. I believe The Fly with Jeff Goldblum was the first of the genre to gain a real audience, but others followed. Aliens in particular scared the bejesus out of me when I finally saw it in my twenties. An alien creature, born and living inside the human body, waiting to burst out and grow into a full-blown killing machine. I can't stand body horror movies. It's always a parasite, or an alien life form, or some type of macabre disfigurement or transformation of the body that doesn't as much scare as it does give me the creeps.

Needles are like that to me. The TAH too, if I'm being honest. Someone is putting something unnatural into my body, and it stays there, and I can't control what it's doing. I can even see where it goes into my body, feel the pinch in the wound when I twist too far in the wrong direction, or raise my arm too far above my head. It's a special kind of psychological horror that is worse to me than fright. It's a daily battle to accept that I have to live with this for now, put it aside, and get on with my day.

Swan caths were a whole Mt. Everest full of body horror for me. Every six weeks or so, it started with the IV, then a bit of sedation, but sometimes not.

I was even giving the phlebotomist team at Hershey Med Center quite the challenge. As my heart was thickening, my vascular system, like my other organs, was getting slipshod profusion. My veins had become small, wiry, and hard to find. Of course, this only exacerbated my needle-phobia, because now, it was highly unlikely for nurses to actually "get the stick" on the first try. Which meant pulling the needle out, setting up again, and taking a second shot. After a while, it became a third. I was enduring the sticks better, but my internal squeamishness had not subsided one iota. At some point along the way, I don't even know how or when, I'd just decided that this was part of it, and I had to endure it to get to the other side. "This is just part of it," became an oft quoted phrase between Christie and me.

I don't remember when I first ended up with Dave drawing my blood. He was just a random tech in the outpatient clinic to me. I'd seen him before, but he'd never drawn my blood. It had to have been a typical Wednesday morning, before the TAH, in the middle of all the swans cath years. He's gangly guy, bouncy and casual. The only person in the place not wearing scrubs. Before I knew he'd gotten me, he'd threaded the vein, gotten all three tubes, and was out. I'd never even felt the needle go in.

I determined that we should become instant friends.

It became a matter of course for the girls in reception to either bump me forward or push me back without my asking, so that I had Dave every time for blood draws. It got down to three times a week before the TAH. By then, Dave knew my whole story, and I knew his. I'd update him on how the family was doing, he'd keep me up to speed on the vacation cabin he was building out in Berks county. He started having to prep my arms, and eventually my hand with hot packs for several minutes before trying to stick me. Once he'd missed a few times, we started talking about getting access through the veins in my legs or feet. Despite his struggles during this time, the song Needlebeast has nothing to do with him. He is the exception.

In the blur surrounding the TAH surgery, I finally had a PICC line placed in my arm (the same one Rich showed the EMT). It's a small tube that's inserted into the soft underside of the arm, just below the bicep. Mine had two capped leads that hung on the outside, while the other 12 inches or so followed the vein as near to the heart - now TAH - cavity as they could get it. Two leads so one could be used to draw blood, the other for administering medicine quickly if need be. That couldn't get mixed up or it had to be pulled and exchanged for a new line. Both were taped down, secured to my arm and kept occluded by a large, clear bandage. The dressing had to be changed once a week and had been since the TAH was implanted.

The PICC site cleaning proved to be more painful than the TAH site cleaning, or any needle. I had the great fortune of finding a nurse in the cancer suite, Jen, who was both fast and efficient, and able to carry out the cleaning without causing much pain at all. Later, once I was living on the HVI, Fred from the PICC team would come to my room once a week to do it. I looked forward to seeing him, but not to the cleaning. It involved creating a sterile field around my arm, both myself and the technician wearing masks so as not to accidentally sneeze or breathe directly on the site itself. The two leads had to be moved around, so the actual insertion site could be cleaned with Chlorhexidine, the chemical that Perry warned me would "burn like Satan's piss." He forgot to mention that Satan also had a bladder infection. Every week I'd try not to writhe and pull away from the biting, blistering sensation as Fred wiped the area down, apologizing the whole time. The site ached for a couple of days after if I didn't immediately take Tylenol, and sometimes even if I did. Eventually we realized Fred could just use iodine instead, which left a sickly orange stain behind, but didn't burn like...well, you know.

The initial PICC line insertion is bad, nothing like the A-line they placed going into the TAH surgery, but to me, awful in both the physical and psychological sense. Because the vein where it's placed goes straight to the heart, everyone is fully suited and masked, and a drape is put across my head, forcing me to turn my head the opposite direction. I don't think I've even once in all of this watched a needle actually go into my body. I do well enough to just get through it each time without vomiting. But it helps me to be aware of the other person's movements and have some sense of when something is going down. With the PICC line, I have only my ears to clue me in, because I can only see the sheet covering my head.

The first time the PICC was placed, the tech told me, "It doesn't hurt at all - we give some lidocaine to numb the area, so you won't feel it."

Lidocaine needs to penetrate deep into the muscle; the needles are long, and the shots are painful. They burn and freeze all at the same time, and it feels like the needle is going all the way to the bone. But the local anesthesia doesn't help much when the actual PICC sheath pierces the flesh of my arm. I can feel almost everything, and even worse, though it doesn't hurt on the inside, I can distinctly feel the pressure of it being forced into my arm and through the vein - I can feel it inside of me, working its way up my arm and into my chest as the tech watches on ultrasound to guide him. It's unnerving.

This line has to be pulled and moved to a different arm every three months, so I had it done three times while on the TAH. The second time, I got the same line: "It doesn't hurt. We give you lidocaine."

"Oh," I said. "So, when did you have yours?"

This was met with a puzzled expression from the nurse. "A PICC line? I've never had one."

"Well then, you wouldn't really know, would you?"

She's taken aback that I would question her word. "We always give lidocaine at the site, so you really shouldn't feel it."

I grabbed the bottom of my gown and yanked it up to my neck, exposing underwear, the gruesome TAH insertions, and the still healing scar that ran the length of my sternum.

"If you don't mind, I'm going to keep my own council on what hurts and what doesn't. This," I said politely, patting the TAH dressing with the other hand, "hurts. But this," I say pointing to the PICC sheath that will house the new tube," hurts. Like. Hell. It's my right to have sedation. I. Want. The. Sedation. Or you can take me back to my room."

Self-advocacy, kids. It's the only way to Fly. Especially when you do it Frequently.

She was irritated, but I got a good dose of Fentanyl and fell asleep shortly after the lidocaine shots went in. But Nurse Never Had a PICC got me back good by ignoring the warning to put the special skin barrier between me and the bandage to avoid blisters, and within six hours, I had to have the dressing changed. Just in that time, I'd already developed several raw spots that had to be treated with the Chlorhexidine, complete with Fred apologizing and me wishing leprosy on Nurse Never Had a PICC through gritted teeth.

Needles, swans caths, IV's, dressing changes, PICC lines...I never got used to any of this, I just endured it, dreading it each time I had to have something done. Down the road, I had the displeasure of undergoing the grandmother of all needle sticks – the dreaded lumbar puncture, or spinal tap, as it's called. But that's a story for another time.

***

In the present, I'm still in the ER, but the nausea and vertigo have finally subsided, and Dave finally comes down to the ER to get the blood cultures; nails it on the first try. They go to the lab and the results come back.

Nothing.

A virus? A one-hour stomach bug? A device anomaly?

"You need to stay here," Dr. Brehm tells me the next day in his thick, German accent. "We don't know what happened. But if it happens again, you need to be here."

Thanks to Brennan, we've already made this decision, back before the surgery, in the gazebo just outside. I've been home for a bit. We'd hoped it would be normal, but it's been incredibly taxing. If I'm admitted, Christie's still running back and forth to the hospital every single day one way or the other. But I'm also getting that coveted 1A time. And just like chronic criminals who say they "know how to jail," thanks to all my swans cath stays and Perry, I "know how to HVI."

My birthday is a bitter-sweet affair. Cologne that I won't wear later because it reminds me of the hospital, and kitchen tools that I won't be able to use until…after.

And that's the reality that settles in during that first week. I'm not going home, until. All the moving, all the roads driven, all the medications and procedures, juggling finances, the hoping and wondering have come down to this.

This is it. The last stretch. I leave here with a new heart, or I leave in a body bag. Maybe even both.

I lobby aggressively for Perry's old room. Room 1170, at the end of the hall. It's the biggest, the most private, the quietest. A tan, brick wall is the only view, but the window just outside the room overlooks a picnic area. It's close to the fridge in the food room. I think the patient that currently inhabits it gets sick of my lingering near the door with questions about how he's doing and when he's headed home. I tell the nurses how good he looks at every chance, and that by my diagnosis, he's all good and ready to leave.

The second week, Carolyn gets me moved in to 1170. It takes a bit of maneuvering, but Tyler and I recreate Perry's layout; bed against the wall, chair turned to the TV. A card table for board games in the middle, Xbox connected, guitar on a stand in the corner. By the third week, I've ordered a magnetic hotplate, a compact convection oven, and a plug-in travel cooler from Amazon. I subscribe to Home Chef's boxed meal service and start cooking for myself. No way I'm going to survive here for any length of time without decent food. If there's anything I've learned, good food is medicine for the soul. Good wine, too, but I don't see sneaking any of that onto the premises. I have my guitar, and my laptop; if only there were room for more beds, so Christie and the boys could stay nights sometimes. I feed the nurses as often as possible to stave off complaints about breaking protocols. Don't ask, don't tell.

Chapter 12

Hope Springs Eternal

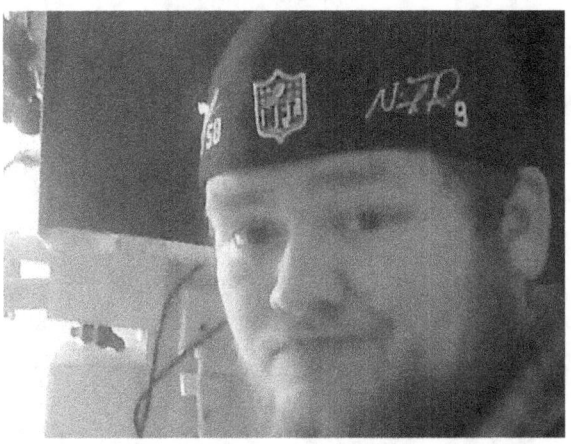

*There always was a reason to believe
The stories I heard, the lines never blurred,
the reason that I couldn't see
Hanging on, the soldier's song, today I have nothing to say
But between the lines, I thought I might find,
a truth that was one and the same*

***And hope springs eternal here
Even though we're all wasting away
Hope springs eternal here
We doubt and we pray, hoping that someday... maybe***

Conversations from Room 1170

There always was a reason, not to hear
The good with the bad, the smoke that we grab,
attrition of marching for years
Waiting for, our miracle, the story we tell will be true
But back in my bed, the lies hurt my head,
I know we won't all make it through

And all of this time is just passing,
while everyone else just belongs,
When I have been frozen and melted for years,
and held by the sleeve for so long
Maybe today, maybe we're gone with the tide
Maybe tomorrow, I won't feel like I've already died.

There always was a reason not to see
The stories I heard, the lies so absurd,
the reason I could not believe
Hanging on, the survivor's song, I have only myself to blame
Down for the count, I never found,
the truth that would make everything okay

I'm getting messages from Perry's sister, Sam every day now.

"Perry's having a lung biopsy tomorrow."

Nothing for a few days. He's on the other side of the unit, across the outer hall where I can't go without a nurse. I've been told it's best that I don't go down there anyway. Perry's still in an induced coma and I don't need the stress. Sam finally messages me a few days before the end of January.

"He has lymphatic cancer."

A few days later, I start getting PM's from Sam around noon. They've been called during the night to the hospital because his team know it's time. I still don't really believe it, though I can tell that everyone's been trying to prepare me for it for weeks now.

Still, he'll tolerate no sappiness from me. Not right now. He is a walking, breathing, no bullshit zone. You have one chance to figure that out because there is no second. End stage HCM survivors can be like that. If I buy into the notion that this might beat him, he'll just ridicule me later.

My memories of that day are blurred. I drink an inordinate amount of ginger-ale because vomiting makes the alarms on my TAH pump go crazy. I don't walk around the unit at all. It's so quiet. No one is talking or making eye contact. We all know what's coming. It feels like the world is holding its breath. Death sticks his head into the room and gives me a salute. He has no business with me today, but just wants to make sure I know he's around. I want to cross the hall to sit outside of his room. But the staff is struggling enough as it is. They don't need trouble from me on top of it.

I get the text from Sam around midnight.

"He's gone."

About two minutes later Krista and Allison knock at my door. The HVI has fallen victim to Perry's particular brand of curmudgeonly cynicism, far too developed for a 19-year-old. They've let him worm his way past their professional exterior and that purposeful distance they're taught to keep between themselves and their patients. And now they're going to pay for it. It's obvious on Krista's face when the door opens. She repeats the words of Sam's text, monotone and numb. She's not been crying. I don't either. Allison leaves, but Krista pulls up a chair and we sit there in silence together for some ten minutes, intruders in the room that had been his home for nearly a year before. There's nothing to say really, to rage against or remember. Perry's shenanigans and hit-and-run wisdom are too close yet to be memories. She leaves without a word, back to attending other patients who aren't him, will never be him. I sleep that night like I haven't in weeks. I've finally exhaled.

How long will I look for him in familiar places, pick up my phone, expecting that text to be from him? Maybe forever. His words are in my head, and I will parrot them back when I talk to people about organ donation, when I lobby for long-term care patients and advocate for early HCM screenings and treatment, later, when I can. All the original things I have to say have been replaced by the words of a ninteen-year-old who said them better than I, and not because he was preparing a speech or blog post. He was just observing his predicament and his place in the world with an eye for detail and an objectivity that I know, even now at forty-seven years of age, I will never attain.

"You just have to stare it in the face. Don't say you're not terrified. We're all terrified, but damned if I'm going to let it know." He wasn't talking about death. He was talking about everything leading up to it. That was our shorthand. He meant HCM, the TAH, the transplant, the recovery. And UNOS. Always UNOS, both savior and executioner.

"It doesn't matter to you or me whether we actually make it or not. We just have to not lose ourselves along the way." He figured dying was the easy part – everyone does it whether they're good at it or not. The hard part was getting there intact. And he did. Not perfectly. Not with the grace that we all fool ourselves into thinking we'll have at the end. But he ended well. Better than anyone could have expected of him, considering the short time in which he had to figure out how to do it. Would that I have a modicum of the stuff he was made of when my time comes.

The next morning, his mother asks me to write the eulogy. It takes me the better part of the day, and I'm emotionally drained afterwards.

Hey Perry,

Dave Johnson

I know this was an open-ended conversation and we picked up the threads from time to time, but now I have to close it and I don't know how to. I talk more than you anyway, so I guess it's only fair. But we had to talk about this, right? It's something that's really too hard to talk to your family or close friends about - not really talk. Too much baggage. It was easier when we didn't know each other so well at the beginning - it was a safe place to say things we wouldn't dare say to other people. Then it got harder because it's safe to talk about dying with a passing stranger. But once you know them, you don't want to think about it anymore. They go from being a statistic to being a friend, and it's impossible for us to imagine a friend becoming a statistic. It's easier to imagine it happening to ourselves, because we know in our hearts that we are not immortal. We know what it feels like for everything to spin out of control. But that friend? That's the guy who won't ever let it get him. I don't know how. Maybe because he's been through so much, that you come to suspect he's superhuman. So, I have to confess, I simply overestimated your immortality. I still can't think of you as anything other than indestructible. Everyone did. And that miscalculation shows on the faces of everyone here today. I hear the miscalculation in the quiet that has overtaken the HVIC unit. The nurses are trying really hard to work, but we're all a bit lost. Krista's a mess. A few people won't make eye contact with me. Kat is putting on a brave face, but I can hear it in her voice. Everyone is either numb or trembling

You were already out of it when they admitted me on the 16th. They moved me down to 1170, or as we call it here on the HVIC, "Perry's room." They didn't know whether to put me here or in 20, right next to where you've been since the day after Christmas. I think this room was the wiser course, because I would have likely tried to sleep in the chair next to you or refused to move from the hallway outside your door, if my IV cable and TAH hose would have reached that far. So here I am, sitting in your chair, using your TV and bathroom. Of course, I'm keeping it cleaner than you did because you're a slob, dude. Still, it's weird, your stuff not being here. Even weirder that you're not in here when I come back from a walk, cussing at Ryan or Tyler for creaming you in Madden. I feel like I'm violating your privacy somehow.

Remember that time you put the Ghost Pepper sauce in Adam's coffee? He was sick for a whole day, but we were laughing about it the other night. It was a good prank. Sean's not here anymore, but I'm sure he'd laugh about the apple incident too. Lori defected back to the float pool but every time I see her she wants to do a skin assessment. Glad you got such a kick out of my victimization. Jerk. A lot of people are gone now, which is pretty much your fault. They can't come in this room anymore, and they can't focus without the thump of your Freedom Driver as you try to dictate which nurse you'll have or bugging them to walk over to the Slushie machine in the Children's hospital with you. They've either left or moved to other units because they screwed up and got emotionally involved. Impossible not to. You kind of sucked people in that way.

It just seems like this whole thing should have ended right, ya know? The story of a young guy who struggled with HCM his whole childhood, implanted with a TAH at 18, going on to transplant and having a long, happy life. Because for some reason, those are the only stories people want to hear. They don't want to hear about brain bleeds, bone marrow cancer, ECKMO machines, ventilators, bleeding out, brain damage, transfusions, and then at the end...the good guy loses. You gotta admit, it makes for a really crappy story.

But it's our story, right? The one about private battles fought in P.E. class in jr. high when you couldn't run the laps like everyone else. Hiding out to escape the inevitable pain that will plague you the rest of the day if you do the push-ups. A-fib spinning the room around, and that frantic moment when it feels like someone just dropped a truck on your throat. Waking up in the middle of the night and it really hits you that your life is at the mercy of a machine you don't understand, or even trust. And *trying to breathe through the panic so the alarm doesn't go off. Holding at bay the worry that you could buy it at any time. Watching friends fall away as the drama burns itself out when they realize there may be no end to this. It's okay that they can't finish the story with you, but it's another battle to let them go and not be angry. About making plans for a food truck and an apartment, soccer with the kids, and drum sets, and fantasizing about a normal life on the other side - one you know is unlikely to ever exist because of rejection and biopsies and immuo-drugs and possibly dying from the stupid common cold.*

But you talk about it anyway, and you make plans because it helps you, just for a moment, to believe that there really is life beyond these small rooms filled with needles and tubes and finger pricks and painful dressing changes and PICC line changes. In the end, you fall asleep knowing that you probably shouldn't have talked about it at all, because it just makes you want it more, and there's nothing you can do to make it happen. If there's one thing that HCM transplants like us know, it's to not get your hopes too high. They've been smashed so many times that you don't have the energy to pick up the pieces anymore. It's not a story for TV. But it's our story and it's important because some of the time, we actually won those small battles. And we're the only ones who know how much strength and soul it sucked out of us. And I think it's okay to be proud of surviving the things we did, even if it's just one more measly blood draw.

Remember how on the last episode of Scrubs, J.D. walks out of the hospital doors that last time and has a vision of all the things that might be? Friendships, and family, and happily ever after? And he's at such peace because even though he can't really see into the future, he sees a possible future, and that's enough?

I want that moment. Where I see you living in our spare room, just like we planned, being my trained volunteer in case the TAH malfunctions. And Rich and Brennan not having to carry that weight. Where I see you in your food truck, knocking out that fantastic BBQ Lasagna and all the fusion foods we worked on during my last SWANS cath. I'm working the window between taking orders and there's a big heart painted on the outside of the van. And everyone knows our story - that we fought a war together and came out the other side with all the scars and the lessons that we learned. That you're older and I am wiser. And then we go to the apartment you had your eye on and your girlfriend and Christie meet us there with the boys and you beat us badly at Settlers of Catan and then gloat about it. You're a horrible winner, did I ever tell you that? And the kids pig out on Warheads and Troll Bites because you keep way too much candy around (if they end up with diabetes, I'm totally blaming you). I want that moment, in the middle of normal life, when no one else notices the look we exchange that says we know, between the two of us - we won the war.

But now I'm forced to let go of that moment, and remember this part, with all the tubes and machines and blood, and more needles, and remember every time I look up from my laptop how I came to be in your room. I'm forced to admit that for all the bloody battles we won, that the war was lost. It's not your fault. It's just biology, and sooner or later it gets the better of us all. It's stupid to say it's not fair that it got you sooner - that's obvious. The hardest part for me will be holding myself back from trying to make sense of it. Because no one can, and anyone who thinks they can is a damned liar. We talked a lot about that too.

I can say with a lot of conviction that I'm going to win my war. Maybe in that way, it'll feel a little like we both won, somehow. Probably not. Then again, we both know that no matter how strong our will is, and how righteous our determination, we are at the mercy of biology. And it's nothing personal - it's just doing the job Mother Nature gave it to do. There are hopes and prayers, but we also both know that in this environment, there are way more tragedies than miracles. We've seen enough of both. I allowed myself to hope for a miracle, though I've never seen anything to make me believe in such a phenomenon. I'd hoped the third-hand anecdotes were true, that maybe I would have one of those unbelievable stories about you. But we don't get to pick our stories.

I'll stay away from the fish in the cafeteria, like you said, and use the TV for my Xbox whether they like it or not. I'll check in on Jamie every day for you (I've been doing it the last two weeks if that makes you feel any better) and even try to get her to eat real food when I can. Tommy came by today to check in on you like he always does, and to say goodbye. Nearly everyone did. I'm giving Adam a lot of crap on your behalf and when I see Sean, I'll tell him you said hello. I'll stay in touch with Mudge and Terri too. But I don't promise to stay here long. Eventually the HVIC will be absent of me and Jamie as well, one way or another, and life will move on until most of us forget each other. If I do come out of this alive, and get to tell my story, it will be partly because, despite your age, you made me face reality at some pivotal moments when I almost blew it. And because even though it was a risk, you determined to finish the war, win or lose. Sometimes it's just the fighting that counts and you should get a medal for that. I'm glad we got to fight a little bit together. I expect the air is easier to breathe now, and there are no more machines to keep you from flying.

Clear skies to you, my brother.

***

Angie tries to get me out for the memorial service, but I thought it wouldn't be a good idea to go (and insurance would use it as a reason not to pay for me to come back). Me with the 'thump thump' of the TAH, ringing out in the silence of a packed church, and worst-case scenario, if I were to fall apart, the alarms would start going off because of the staggered breathing. And the last thing I want to do was sit in a church service where some well-meaning priest tells us all about God's plan and how Perry's in a better place now. No one ever wants to address my theological questions about suffering and death in this life, and I sure didn't want to break any more fingers trying to budge that boulder in the middle of a memorial service. Luther and Calvin had no answers, so I doubt any mere mortal is going to wow me with some new revelation that second year seminary students aren't already squabbling over at South-southeastern-west Bapticostal Seminary or wherever the hell (probably in Dallas). Stow it, guys. Even Adrian Rogers admitted to struggling with it. What hope do you or I have?

We go to the impromptu memorial at the hospital chapel instead, but only a few people from the HVI come because it's in the middle of shift (everything is in the middle of shift for nurses, one way or the other). Perry's mom and sisters are there, as well as his dad. He pays me a visit on an emotional - and I suspect chemical - high, after he heard my eulogy at the service. I'm nice as I can be, but I know Perry's opinion of him, and I don't think he realizes how dangerous it is at that moment for anyone who's crossed Perry to cross paths with me. Good thing I'm attached to a life-sustaining backpack pump. It's never bad to have grace with people, I just suspect that those who give it out freely either kickbox or drink copiously afterwards to let the anger out, or keep it in, respectively. I'm not in any position to indulge in either.

***

I don't think most of us understand how hope works. Humanity has held to it in the darkest of situations, even when they knew it would go unrewarded. Despite the sheet covered bodies that are rolled off the unit every week, and the misery I hear coming from some of the rooms at various times, hope endures. Hope is a foolish thing to hold onto unless you can hold it at arm's length, away from yourself enough to see it in context. It's that small part of me that says I can't stop walking - just in case. The waiting list is slippery, but hope latches onto it, believing there's a way to overcome the very laws of math itself. We know we won't all make it out alive. But someone just might. Maybe Blake or Jamie. Maybe even me.

I've also found that hope is useless at cleaning the hard drive in my brain. Stored there are images I can't black out, no matter how brightly hope shines. Perry bleeding. Dot's last noncommittal shrug. Jamie's daughters standing timidly at the door of this person who used to take care of them. And now James, his dry lips smacking while he whispers to his wife, his blue eyes bulging from a face that looks all but skeletal. The image that plays on a loop is the worst one. I'm standing at the double-doors that lead back to the main hospital, waving and making faces at the boys through the glass, while Christie tries to smile instead of cry. I do anything to make them laugh, and they're still just young enough to give into the silliness. But eventually I have to keep myself from poking my head back around the corner. I know they're waiting there, on the other side of the door, to see if I'll stick my leg out or do something funny just one more time, but they have to get home, and I have to let them go. After I'm sure they've given up and headed for the van, I poke my head around the corner just one more time, hoping maybe they've out-waited me and they're still there, looking. Then I sit in the windowsill looking out at the parking lot for a long time. This is a quiet spot on the HVI at night, and it's just me and the thump of the TAH. I don't think about anything particular. I try not to think. I just need a few moments before I go back to the room that's been filled with games and food and chatter for the last few hours, and hope that this helps. I wonder if Blitzy and Stitch, our dogs, still wonder where I am when they come home without me. I hope they do, but maybe that makes it worse for Christie and the boys. Hope doesn't purge my mind of any of this. It just keeps hitting the play button, over and over.

And yet, it's because of all this that I want to believe that I'll make it. I've never found comfort in the Pollyanna philosophy that if I believe something hard enough, it will come true. While a solid and reliable principle in Disney films and anecdotal church stories, my hard beliefs have always left me disappointed, disillusioned, broke, and scrambling to put out fires. Hope isn't a magic pill that makes me feel better. It's not much more than a bit of fantasy, reminding me what it might be like if I ever have a normal life again. And that has to be enough for now.

I don't know how long I can hold out hope. Perry was still going after fifteen months. I'm prepared to go at least that long. Hope springs eternal, so the saying goes. But hope, like faith is based on evidence, and I've seen little evidence of late that there's much of anything to hope for.

Chapter 13

One Step

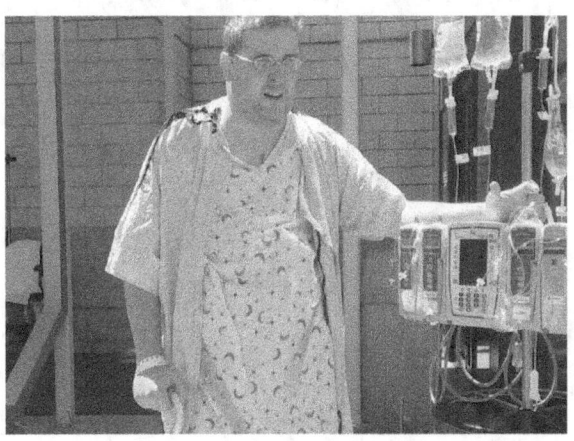

It's not the endless circles, it's the monochromatic scenery
It's not the muscles burning, it's the lie that someday I'll be free
It's not the prison or the prison walls,
it's the carrot at the end of the string
It's not the hand-holding or the way we bleed,
it's the sirens and the bells and the never-ending ringing

One step, one foot in front of the other,
One step, walking in the steps of another

It's not the roller coaster, it's the way my mother smiles at me
It's not the burning changes,
it's the waking dread that won't let me be
It's not the four walls pushing in

Conversations from Room 1170

it's the window with the brickyard view
It's not the mush, the restriction, the sterility,
it's that everyday always brings nothing new

It's not the hope eternal, it's the waiting in our unwashed skin
It's not the guns and the urinals,
it's the way the rules won't let me in
It's all the same, it's all the rain, it's all the sleeping in
The needles, the scopes, my fading hope,
most of all – it's my indifference

One step, another round so I don't smother
One step, wearing out the shoes of my brother

What now?

Walk. Have you walked today? You need to walk.

I don't want to walk. I don't think I can walk anymore. I've been tramping around this same circular path for the better part of two years. The same desks. The same faces. The same pictures on the wall. I don't want to see anyone, and besides, it's like a graveyard out there ever since . . . well . . .

It's strange and comforting to be in Perry's old room. Good memories here, if there's such a thing in this place. I have to stay busy or I start to brood. He lived here for over a year. I'm only into my first month and I'm sick of everything. The empty promises that it will be over soon. The sterile white and grays, the monotony of shift changes, the needles, the batteries, the lifeless brick wall outside my window. I'm tired of staying up too late and sleeping in. I'm tired of it not mattering whether it rains, or snows, or is a nice warm day. What does it matter? I'm trapped in here at a controlled 72 degrees and nothing beyond these walls affects me. Most of all, I'm sick and tired of the walking. All the walking, around and around and around, like some kind of horse in a coral.

I try not to look out the windows because it reminds me that there's a world beyond this one. Then there's that voice.

"You need to walk. You're going to end up with a blood clot. You want a stroke? You wanna drown? Get up off your lazy ass and walk. Wussy."

I can't today. I can't. It's just one day.

"It's just one step. You put one foot in front of the other. We've done this a million times. You skip today, it'll be easier to skip tomorrow. Walk. Ten laps."

Five.

"Okay, five, since you're being a girl about it."

I wonder how long this voice is going to be in my head. I sigh and sling the backpack on. When I pull open my door and step onto the hallway, it's like walking into a crypt. No call bells or talking. Everyone is either in a room or with their heads down at the computer. Alex passes me on her way back to her station, eyes red and puffy. Even Larry, the cleaning guy who's become a good friend, has apparently taken the day off to avoid being here. I wish I could call in.

The first left on my never-ending track takes me past Jamie's room. She's sitting on her bed, still unable to walk with her cobbled together assist device, staring out the door. She stirs when she sees me, looks up with a blank expression.

"You okay?" I ask her.

She shakes her head and says in her tiny, raspy voice. "I don't know. I'm indifferent. Does that make me bad?"

"I think we're all bad," I tell her. "I just don't know what we're being punished for."

I stand there in her doorway for a moment. There's nothing else to say.

Conversations from Room 1170

"Where ya going?" she asks when I turn away.

"Walking," I say over my shoulder. "Gotta keep walking."

***

The other reason we walk is because too much sitting around can cause blood clots in your legs. When you start moving around, they can break loose and travel to the brain or lungs. I can deal with an artificial heart. The ultimate terror for me is to be trapped inside my own body while my mind doesn't function right. We check my blood coagulation twice a day for the same reasons we did at home, and it's no hassle with the PICC line; they just screw the syringe head into the threads on the PICC "ports" hanging out of my arm and draw it without a needle. But sometimes they need fresh blood from a fresh site. Like when I have a stroke.

Dan, my nurse for the day whom I've known for two years, comes in to enter my morning vitals - weight, blood pressure, O2 level, etc. - into the computer. I make this easier for them by just doing them myself when I wake up. It's coming up time for my 11 o'clock pills.

Apparently, Dan informs me that he's going to run to the caf and grab a bite, then bring my pills in when he gets back. Apparently, I also ask him to grab me a few BBQ chicken wings, since that's a once a week thing at the caf, and one of the only barely edible things there.

The next thing I remember is Tina, the device tech, checking numbers on the Big Machine. I've been transferred back to it from the Freedom Driver. I'm lying in bed, asking her what happened. Then a flash of Dan saying, "Dammit, Dave, I'm not answering that again. It's hospital protocol!" Then Christie standing over the bed. I'm elated to see her because she worked last night and should be sleeping, but she's here to see me! "You should be sleeping," I tell her. "Why are you here?"

Another blurry moment and then Dave, the one-shot wonder- is squatting next to my bed with two bottles that I know are for holding blood cultures.

"Dave!" I say. "Hey, man! Thanks for coming up." I have no idea why he's there.

"Hey buddy," he says, "We gotta get some blood cultures. Just hang tight. I've got you."

"Sure," I say. I may have gone to sleep or things just got fuzzy again. I knew something was wrong, but once I saw Dave, I knew it would be okay. Dave has me. Dave's always got me.

Then I remember Christie standing over the bed telling me to name all the Rush albums in order. It's a little thing I do when I'm coming out from under sedation. One of my favorite bands, Rush, has a long and distinguished discography, and I know if I can go all the way through it in my head, I'm close to lucidity again. If I really want to gauge where I am, I work my way through Chris Squire's bass rigs through the years. Squire played bass for the band Yes through their forty-plus year career, and he is far and away one of the most important musicians in my personal musical development and journey. I've obsessively studied him for nearly twenty-five years, to the point that I know exactly what model and year of instrument he used on each Yes recording, along with his respective amplifier setup, and any pedals and effects he may have used. If any of this varied from one album or tour to the next, it's locked into my memory banks and I can recall it faster than I can recall mine or my children's birthdays or social security numbers. It's a sickness.

But Rush is easy. "The self-titled album was first, of course," I say, prepared to breeze through this. "But we don't count that one sometimes because it's the only one with the original drummer, John Russey. Once Neal replaced him, there's been *Fly by Night*, released on the exact day of my birth in 1971, I want it noted. Then *Caress of Steel, 2112, All the World's a*

Stage, which was live. That was the first five album cycle. Then, *A Farewell to Kings . . . Permanent Waves, Moving Pictures, Exit-Stage Left* . . . no wait. I've missed one."

This is inconceivable to me. "*2112, A Farewell to Kings, All the World's a Stage . . . Permanent Waves*. No. What comes after *Farewell*?" My stomach drops. I realize something really bad has happened. The loss of time, the blurry memory of the day. Christie is here. I'm not on the Freedom Driver. Dave was here. And now I remember Dr. Falcuchi and Brehm being here. It's blurry but I remember seeing them. Dr. Hight was here asking me what day it was, and Falcuchi wanted me to tell him who had passed away the day before. George Martin, the fifth Beatle, I know now, but I remember not being able to tell him at the time. Oh God. How could I not remember George Martin dying? I worship the man. I cried when I heard the news, shut myself in my room, and listened to The Beatles for the rest of the day. I was devastated. How did I not remember that? Even worse, how could I not recite the Rush discography?

"It's not just short term," Christie tells someone over her shoulder. "He's missing some long-term too."

"Well, you wouldn't be able to tell from that..."

Christie's voice is fierce. "This man has trouble remembering his own mother and father's birthday. He barely remembers his own. But he can recite the Rush discography in his sleep. He can tell you what record label they were all on and what date, not the year, but the DAY they were released, and probably what number they charted on that day. That is hard-core long-term memory for him. He's missing both."

"What happened to me?" I whisper.

"You had a TIA," Christie says. She's upbeat, but I can tell she's scared. "It's like a mini-stroke. You lose short-term memory. Maybe some long-term, but not usually."

The commotion dies down once I can carry on a lucid conversation. Christie settles herself in my chair and dozes off, but I can't sleep. I'm wide awake, double-checking my memories, year by year, quizzing myself on things that should be on my internal hard drive. I eventually try the Rush albums again.

"*Hemispheres*!" I shout out. Christie, wakened from sleep, lets out a startled yelp.

"*All the World's a Stage, HEMISPHERES*," I continue, "*Permanent Waves, Moving Pictures, Exit-Stage Left, Signals, Grace Under Pressure!*" I'm on a roll now. If I can get through this, maybe it means I haven't lost long-term memories. "*Hold Your Fire, Power Windows, A Show of Hands, Presto, Roll the Bones, Counterparts, Test for Echo* . . . um, um . . . *Different Stages, Vapor Trails, Snakes and Arrows, Working Men, Clockwork Angels*!"

She calls Dan back to the room.

"What year is it?" Dan asks.

"2016, Obama's in the White House, yada yada. Hey Dan."

"Oh. Now I'm Dan," he says with mock disgust.

"You were calling him Ben," Christie says. "That's how he knew something was wrong."

"I brought your chicken wings, and you were mad because you didn't want chicken wings. You clear as day asked me for chicken wings, and I brought you chicken wings and you were acting weird and kept calling me Ben," Dan says.

I have no memory of this.

"After about the fourth time I was getting mad, then I realized you weren't right."

"That's why you're here," I say to Christie. My mind is reeling now. How can I have gone through an entire afternoon, talking and interacting with people and only remember bits and pieces? I've already told Christie, I can live with paralysis, loss of speech, or even blindness. But I wouldn't want to live without my mind. That would be a living death that I want no part of. Is this a taste of what people with delirium or Alzheimer's experience?

"That's why I'm here," Christie says, "Every time I came near the bed for about four hours, it was like the first time you'd seen me."

"And I swear to God," says Dan, entering info into the computer, "if you'd asked me why I couldn't just get blood cultures from your PICC line again, I was going to punch you out."

"You didn't use blood from the PICC for cultures, did you?" I asked alarmed, "you can't do that - you need a clean stick."

That gets a weary laugh from everyone in the room.

"I kept telling you that," says Dan. "About the thirtieth time you asked why we couldn't just get blood from the PICC, I told you to shut up, that it was hospital protocol."

"You kept repeating yourself," Christie says. "You asked Tina what was going on so many times she wanted to choke the life out of you."

By the time the sun goes down, I can even remember all of Chris Squire's gear again. Unfortunately, I can also still remember other things I wish I couldn't. And for the life of me, I still don't remember much of anyone's birthdays or anniversaries.

Once the team feels like it's safe, they change me back to the Freedom Driver. We always wait for Tina to do this, along with Dr. Brehm or Pabst. Tina and I have a love/hate relationship I exasperate her with questions about arcane TAH details that she can't answer. She deals primarily with LVADs. It doesn't help that Brian, Mudegman, and I have made an art of harassing her. I've been through this switch over a half dozen times now and the fear has worn off. They count down – '3-2-1' – then disconnect the drive lines from the heart and quickly attach the ones from the already running Freedom Driver. I wait a second as Tina fiddles with the safety ties, then grab my chest and start making horrific gasping sounds from deep in my throat. Tina's flipping out, double checking the pump, the connections, and the driver readings, but Brehm sees me smile and starts laughing out loud. Tina finally catches on and starts slapping me on the arm.

"What's the matter with you?!" she shouts.

"Hey!" I say, trying to dodge, "I'm on the transplant list!

"You're on the shit list!" she snarls. Everyone in the room is cracking up. Poor Tina. If there's a practical joke to be made, she'll inevitably be the target. But she loves us. Kind of.

No harm done, I go back to whatever amounts to normal life on the HVI. I've scared everyone good, and none of the docs know what caused it, or if it will happen again. My main cardiologist, Eric Popjes, has surrendered me to Dr. Brehm and the intensivist team for the duration of the TAH implant, but he comes by every few weeks to check on me. Always with a giant cup of Au Bon sweet iced tea, which he knows I crave, but don't really need because of my blood sugar and fluid restriction. He has a habit of tapping on the glass and waving the tea at me anytime he's around, just to antagonize me. Today he's hanging around after his shift to see how I'm doing. I ask him if there's anything I can do to keep from having another stroke. Anything more serious than the one from the day before, and I'm off the waiting list for who knows how long.

"Yeah," he answers darkly. "Get a real heart."

"That's your job," I shoot back. The conversation in Room 1170 moves on to our hopes for the next Star Wars movie.

***

The pediatric TAH is finally approved, and Jamie gets hers implanted in late February. They have to keep putting her back onto the big machine because the alarms on the Freedom Driver keep going off for unexplained reasons. When they finally get it to work, I take her first lap around the hall with her, in Perry's stead. Neither of us talk about it, but the weight of the loss is heavy at moments like these.

When we get back to her room, she sits on the bed, winded. I resume my normal place in the doorway.

"You okay?" I ask her.

"Tired. I can't remember when I wasn't tired."

We're silent for a while. It's the first time we've hung out since Perry's passing, him being the thing we had in common. I've been cooking for her, trying to make her eat, but she's picky, and Perry found ways to work around that. He was also way more insistent than me. I've been trying to fill those shoes, but I'm not as good at forcing people to do things they don't want to. He'd made it into an art form. I could tell she was losing weight.

"If this doesn't work, I'm not going to let them try it again," she tells me.

"What, just lay there and let whatever happens happen?"

She shrugs. "How long am I going to keep dragging the girls through this? My mom's about to have a nervous breakdown." She takes a long pause. "I'm just so tired."

"You'll feel better the more you walk," I promise her. "It helps your head to work right."

She laughs. "My head's never worked right. Besides, look at how much time I've lost. My girls don't even know me. Every time they leave, I think it'll probably be the last time I see them. It's like I've already died, everyone's just visiting the corpse, like you do at the funeral home."

"That's you. They don't think of it like that. Once you're out, they'll know you again. You'll catch up and it will be better. You're guaranteed not to make it if you just sit around here and wait for it to happen."

She hasn't looked at me the entire conversation, but she does now. Her eyes are red and it occurs to me that in all of this, I've never seen her cry.

"If he didn't make it, what chance do I have?"

I know it's partly the junkie talking. People who've abused drugs feel like they don't deserve an organ, because of what they've done. Which is an entirely social construct with no basis in sound ethical practice or philosophy, but Jamie isn't one to have those kinds of conversations. It's not the first time I've heard this kind of talk from people in her situation, and it won't be the last.

* * *

Dr. Brehm slides into my room one day, a bit sheepish, which is counter to his abrupt German manner. I've trained almost everyone else to knock and started putting big signs on the door after the second time a group of docs walked in with me standing with my pants around my ankles. Dr. Brehm will never be trained to knock. He is Dr. Brehm.

"I was wondering if you might do something for me," he asks cautiously.

"Depends. You've asked me to do some pretty weird things lately," I say, motioning to the Freedom Driver.

He chuckles, a rare gift from him. He's distracted for a moment by the weekly cartoon I draw on my white board. Everything from me defending my food in the breakroom fridge with a rifle and barbed wire, to Mark leaving my room with hundreds of needles sticking out of him after asking for more blood.

"There is a TAH patient. James. Do you know him?"

I figure I know all the TAH patients - there was Perry, Jo, Blake, Sherri, now Jamie, me...and that's it. James must be a new guy.

"Haven't met him yet."

"He's been here a while," Brehm says. This sounds weird to me. Why wouldn't I know him? TAH patients usually gravitate toward one another pretty quickly. We follow the sound of the thumping. "He's depressed and wants to give up. Maybe you could just talk to him. It might help him to see you up and around and doing well."

I've no idea what he means by this, but I have Kat take me down to his room on the other wing of the unit. I'm expecting someone like me, a TAH patient, either with a Freedom Drive in a backpack, or sitting in bed hooked up to the big machine.

James is something completely different. He's attached to the big machine, but he's prone in the bed, hooked up to all the same wires and tubes I remember from my TAH surgery. An NG tube is taped to his scabbed nose and his fingernails are crusted with dried blood. If Perry looked like a shell of himself, James looks like a phantom of a man, pale and emaciated. His wife hovers over the bed, and he whispers in her ear.

"He appreciates you coming," she says with a weary smile. I'd foolishly assumed that I'd seen every stage of exhaustion on Christie's face, but the circles under her eyes, and her anxious expression makes her look ten years older than she probably is.

"Hi, James, I'm Dave," I say directly to him. I kick into pastor mode. Poker face. Don't show any sign of the horror you feel, and talk directly to the patient, even if you're told they can't hear you. But James is cognitive, awake in this freak show of tubes, artificial implants, liquid food, foley catheters, and pain. It reminded me of that scene in The Matrix where Neo wakes in the real world, in the tank, connected to a dozen tubes and wires. "Dr. Brehm said you passed a big milestone today."

"He's come off continuous dialysis, they pulled the tubes this morning," she says.

"How long were you on that?"

"Ever since the TAH surgery," his wife supplies. "About nine months now."

I know my poker face is faltering. It has to be. Nine months? I vividly remember the intense pain I suffered the days following my TAH implant. The incessant, cold ache in my back from laying in the same position alone was enough to make me feel like I must be in some sterile version of hell those nights. He's been laying here like this for nine months? Dr. Brehm didn't bother to share that little tidbit with me.

"That's a big step," I say. "You've gotta be tired, man. Hopefully they can switch you over to the Freedom Driver pretty soon and we'll be walking the loop together out here."

Because you have to walk. "*Walk or drown,*" Perry says in my head. The only reason James hadn't yet, (presumably) is the NG tube in his nose and most likely a water ration that made prison camps look generous. The thirst must be enough to drive a person insane.

She leans down for another whispered exchange. As she stands up, they both have watery eyes. "He wants to know if you ever felt like just giving up."

The man is staring me straight in the eyes. What is he asking me here? If it's okay to give up? If he's a coward if he does? My next words better be right, because he's watching me closely. He'll know if I'm lying.

Conversations from Room 1170

What do I tell him, Perry?

No bullcrap.

"Every day," I say. "Every damn day, James." The tears well up in my eyes too and I can't say much more. The three of us are alone in the room now that the nurse has left, two dead men and one of their angels. And we all know the truth. My old friend, Death, is right there in the room with us. Waiting. Never interfering, never passing judgement. Just waiting. Maybe he has an appointment with James today, maybe with me. But we all know he's there, and we give him his moment of respect, as all mortals must do when he graces us with his presence. Then he's gone.

I take a deep breath. "I got up this morning, and I wondered what I'm doing here. I've been here for a couple of months now. My wife and two boys are at home."

"We have two girls," his wife says.

I return James's stare. "And I have to ask myself, if I'm dragging them through all this for me, or for them? They'll be broken if I die, but they'll also be able to go on and have a normal life. If I stay in this state for who knows how long, this is their life. It's my wife's life. I've been at this for eighteen years, but only the last six have been really bad. And I weigh that in my mind every day. I could lie to you and tell you it gets easier. But living on the Freedom Driver is hard. Better than what you're doing now, but still hard. And we both know that an eventual transplant isn't a guarantee of anything. For me, I've decided that I'll never know if it's better to just check out and let my family move on with their lives, or to stay and fight in the hope that things will eventually be okay. So, I'm not going to take that into my own hands. I'm just defiant enough against God or Death or whatever you want to call it that I feel like, 'if you want me, you have to come get me yourself. I'm not doing your job for you, you lazy bastard!'"

His wife laughs, and James closes his eyes, squeezing out tears. He nods his head a few times and sighs, which causes him to tremble a bit.

"All I can tell you is, you've got a family who wants you around, so you don't have much say in it, right? And you're past a lot of bad stuff now that the perpetual dialysis is done. We need to get you up and walking."

He whispers a thank you and I pat his arm. I see the look on his face - he should be able to shake my hand, but he can't even do that. His eyes say the same thing I feel about a dozen times a day.

What have I been reduced to?

Outside, Mike walks me back to my wing. I bump into the food room and grab a can of Ginger-Ale, then bullet to my room and close the door. On my way to the bathroom I choke down a piece of Reed's ginger candy to settle my stomach and take a swig of the Ginger-Ale. It doesn't help much. I sit on the toilet and dry heave once, quietly, but force myself to get it under control so the alarms don't go off. Vomiting and dry heaving has become such a normal part of my life the last few years, it doesn't take much at all to get me started. James' predicament is more than enough.

It's night shift and Adam pops in to raid my mini-fridge for anything good and "borrow" a bunch of my Jolly Rancher candies.

"It pisses me off that they asked you to do that," he says, kicking a chair back on two legs.

"Well, he got off the dialysis today, so maybe he'll improve."

Adam just shakes his head. "Dave, he's not leaving here alive. They can't get his blood count right. It'll take him months to learn to walk again even if they can. There's no way he's a candidate for transplant anymore. I doubt he ever will be again.

They shouldn't have taken you down there – you didn't need to see that."

I consider myself pretty savvy at this hospital thing by now, but I'm genuinely stunned. "Why did they?"

"Because they don't want him to give up. Numbers, my friend. It's all about numbers."

In other words, if James dies, it'll be the second TAH patient this year. Jo. Perry. Jamie's outlook isn't so good, and Blake can't even be listed until his liver situation improves. James's death affects their success rate with the TAH. Which affects the program's budget. Which reflects on the Penn State Medical system. It's not that they don't care about any of us. But they can't keep caring for people if they have no funding to help them.

A few days later, I hear that James has refused further treatment. He passes in a day or so. I never see his wife again, and now I even forget what she looks like. But I'll never forget his face. To the world, he's just part of the twenty-two people that died that day waiting for a life-saving organ. To me, he's the face of what could have been. I could just as easily have not recovered from the TAH surgery. But I also know his wife must wonder how it could have been different if he'd just held on a bit longer, if maybe they could have had their life back someday. That's the thing about being neither alive nor dead on an implanted heart. You don't know anything. You just wait.

Chapter 14

Silence is Golden

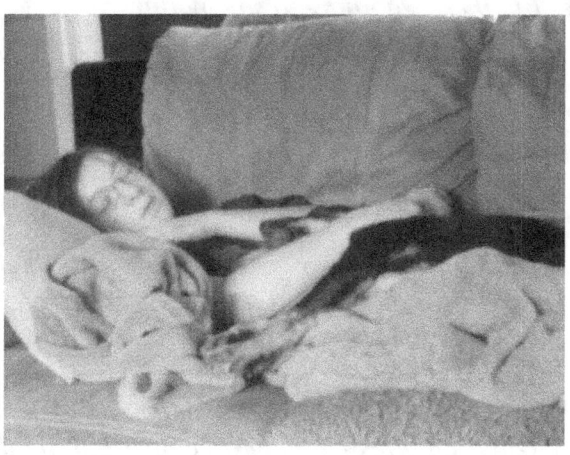

*If I wasn't leaking hope,
If my teeth weren't clenched around the rope,
If I wasn't killing time,
If we knew everything will be fine, fine, fine,*

*But you can't say, I can't say,
With all this confusion trying to have its day,
We can't break through and there's no one to pay,
There's nothing to say, nothing to say,*

**Falling down, silence is golden,
When I drown, I do it out in the open,
Women and the children scream pray to the sky,
But why does everyone avert their eyes?**

Conversations from Room 1170

If anything but limbo would just begin,
If I could just buy into original sin,
As if blood ever fixed a single damn thing,
Like the Ghost is the only thing that ever made me sing,

But I don't know, you don't know,
We're racing down a road few have walked before,
They said one way or another, everybody pays,
But there's nothing to say, nothing to say,

Falling down, silence is golden,
When you pray, the spell is broken,
All the women and children scream look to the sky,
But everyone averts their eyes,

Preaching parrots with their 'everything will work out fine,
Don't whisper those words 'cause they make you shine,
I can't feel this thing they keep talking about,
Can't shut my mind, and so I run my mouth,
Blank stares and a primal sigh,
You can keep it inside but it all comes out in time,

Throughout this entire experience, we've been admonished from every quarter to pray, believe, have faith. Blamed for lack of faith, told I was sick because of something I'd done wrong, some unconfessed sin. Chronically ill people share very similar stories on this count. Everyone has always assumed that they know better than us, that they've correctly diagnosed the problem and found the cure. Prayer, faith, believing God will heal. But he hasn't. And now I'm relying on medicine to survive. I've been relying on it the whole time, but as long as no one can see physical evidence of a sickness, they're happy to believe the root cause is spiritual. I've endured that for about fifteen years. When I announced I'd be implanted with the TAH, the lectures and chiding stopped. I figure most people didn't know what to say.

The majority just started praying a new prayer - for the doctor's wisdom, seemingly oblivious to the fact that the millions of prayers spoken up to this point had made zero impact on my situation, or God's plan, if you choose to view it as such. I still don't know how to talk to folks who think prayer is the cure to everything. I have nothing against prayer, I've engaged in it myself – a lot. But action, not prayer, is what got us out of the situation I was in in Arkansas, and brought us here, to Pennsylvania, where my life will be sustained until I get a heart. And not a single step along the way happened easily, or in answer to a specific prayer. Were that the case, we'd still be living our lives in the Ozarks, and I'd be getting transplanted at the Heart Hospital in Little Rock. And it would have happened four years ago. I could almost make the case that every single thing I've prayed for in this situation has only tipped off a higher power to direct events down the opposite path. This has been tooth and nail every single moment so far. It could be argued that we're somehow being tested for some higher purpose. I'll admit openly I'm failing the test. Mostly, because I'm watching this whole thing eat up my boy's childhood, my wife's physical health, and my own sense of purpose with very little grace or peace. Whatever the test is for, to my mind, it's not worth it.

Nevertheless, most people who believe prayer is the cure-all, will keep believing that until the sick person is buried in the ground, and then move on to the next unfathomable cruelty and continue to pray that it's fixed. Are they praying for God to fix the problem, for him to choose to stop inflicting pain on their loved ones? And when he doesn't, few people seem to wonder why, and continue in the same futile begging that accomplished nothing that last time. Now, everyone tells me I should pray, but when I ask these questions, I'm met with silence. No one wants to make eye contact anymore.

One thing that's strained the limits of my grace (and stretched my ability to keep my mouth shut beyond the breaking point) are the barrage of trite and cliché comments that have been heaped on along the way. Though they've waned noticeably in the face of the TAH, and now Perry's death, they're particularly hard to respond to - or in my case, to respond to kindly. They come from a place of hope and faith, and at the very least, I learn to take them as a sentiment of good will from people who really believe that hope, faith, love, prayer, and other intangibles are more effective than MRI's, assist-devices, or a good surgeon with a sharp scalpel. Most believe that the goodness of God brought these things to be anyway. And I notice this is the same no matter which "God" the person is referencing. Jehovah G-d, Jesus, Allah, Vishnu, Buddha, and (jokingly) The Flying Spaghetti Monster, were all dutifully petitioned to help me survive the TAH surgery. Accordingly, they've all been awarded credit for my survival by their respective believers. But I guarantee no one would be clamoring to take the blame if I hadn't.

Sorting that stuff out is way above my pay grade. I notice that most armchair theologians disappear like roaches when the kitchen light clicks on at midnight if I start crediting their deity for my HCM, which forced me to have the TAH implant in the first place. From their respective followers, I'd hear a lot of theologically heretical explanations about how their particular deity didn't *cause* it, but only *allowed* it. Further questions on my part asking said followers to describe how the two are different, are met with equally fuzzy theology about faith (don't worry, kids. The problem of suffering vexed both Martin Luther and the theological powerhouse, John Calvin. Luther to the point of despair and reportedly, attempted suicide). I could probably help clarify a bit of this, but I've found that trying to actually explain people's beliefs to them serves only to irritate them and send them into a near epileptic state of praising (insert your favorite deity's name here) accompanied by a lot of babbling about "feelings" and "just knowing" (concepts that are a purely Western invention, by the by, and are a completely foreign concept in the theological systems of all three major world religions). I try to not to dismantle the theological framework of well-meaning folk, but sometimes it's like that crooked picture on the wall. You just have to attempt to set it right, even if it falls back crooked. The nail being in the wrong place to begin with is giant worm-can full of spiritual metaphor that's begging to be opened, but I digress.

For a long time now, even before I resigned the ministry, I honestly haven't found much comfort in the idea that God (or the Universe, or Fate, or the other myriad things I've been told to trust in) is in control. The thing I've noticed about all these Powers That Be is that humans never get invited to the board meetings. Gods all have their own agendas which may or may not include keeping me alive. Think about it – you can't really say, "God's going to bring you through this," to me, any more than you could have said it to Perry, or the roughly twenty-two people who died on a transplant waiting list today. Yes, today. That's a lot of people who God didn't bring through this.

It betrays a rather small view of God, and a rather over-inflated perception of just how important I am in the Grand Scheme Of Things. Even the Bible is filled with numerous accounts of God wiping out entire nations for the sake of His plan. My friends in other countries are nodding in agreement, while the American readers are thinking, "But that could never happen to US. We're AMERICANS!" Fact is, no matter what your belief system or theological framework, when it comes to the decisions made by The Powers That Be, none of us hold stock in the company.

In a movie or video game in which the main character faces mortal danger, I always used to assure the kids that nothing will happen to Harry, or Luke, or Iron Man, because, hey, that's the main character. If he dies, there's no game. There's no movie. There's no TV show. So, he can't die. (Well, except in the case of Harry Potter who did die. But that only makes him stronger when he comes back to kick some Death-Eater booty. And there's that Jesus thing too).

If only that were the case in real life. Though I may be the main character in my own story, in Christie's, and even in Rich and Brennan's story until they're older, I'm certainly not the center of any universe anywhere. It took many, many years for me to be convinced of this, but I'm pretty sure I'm not. We all like to think that we're special, that it will work out for *us*. But if everyone is special, then where are the people that it *doesn't* work out for? See, *someone* has to make up that percentage that dies while waiting. Or that dies due to complications. Or a bad match. Or infection. Or rejection. It has to be someone. I have names and faces for the people on that side of the equation. Dot. Jo. Perry. And there will be more. Just so long as it's someone else, right?

But that percentage that doesn't make it? It's made up of people whose friends and families want to believe that they're also at the center of the universe, that God will make an exception for them, that Fate has more for them to do. This is the story of every surviving spouse, child, friend, and parent of someone who dies waiting for a transplant. Twenty-two people, every single day in the U.S. How many more from cancer? How many from some wasting disease you and I can't even pronounce, that will never get funding for research because not enough people die from it?

My sense of humor has become morbid in the extreme, but I'm not by nature a morbid person. Being realistic with myself about the possibilities and my tiny role in the Grand Scheme Of Things really helps me to have a positive outlook on the situation. I've been criticized, and in some cases, cut off by people who were friends at one time, for not having more faith. What they really mean is that I should believe – or have a stronger belief that everything will be okay. And they get frustrated that I don't. Often times, they imply or bluntly state that God will never heal me or save me from death because of this. It's the ultimate "blame the victim" scam, and I've learned to cherish the good memories with those people, but I don't regret that they're no longer in my life.

The word "faith" as it's used in the New Testament is rooted in the Greek word *"pistis."* I won't digress into the etymological dissection a dead language (much as I would enjoy it), but the general idea is that faith is "belief in the direction of evidence." I think that's a great way to approach faith. It's not simply a wide-eyed, vacuous belief that everything is going to come up roses. The idea is that when we see ample evidence that something is true, we should trust that it is.

But that's exactly the reason I honestly don't think faith is going to change a single thing in terms of my outcome. There's a prevailing confusion in many Christian quarters that we should be able to speak things into existence if we have enough faith, as if we're some type of twisted version of the Wonder Twins from the Super Friends cartoon.

"WONDER TWIN POWERS! ACTIVATE! FORM OF… A NEW LIVER!"

Never mind that this is a horrific butchering of both the language and context of the word and the original writer's (probably Paul of Tarsus') intent, this hermeneutical horror is perpetuated by men like Kenneth Copeland, the Oral Roberts Family crime ring, Joel Osteen, Joyce Meyers, and a slew of others who make money by preying on the sick and the old. In other religions it's known as "positive self-talk" or "positive verbal energy." This is closely tied to the so-called "prosperity gospel" in America where folks have been duped into believing that being rich and healthy is possible for anyone who believes hard enough. Hello, Mr. Copeland? The 99% would like a word with you. People who believe this stuff aren't bad – they're just wrong. Unless they're getting rich off it and don't care. Then they're most definitely both bad and wrong.

Anyone with even a remedial knowledge of history or religious literature knows that an overwhelming majority of the evidence speaks to death being part of life, God (or the gods, if you prefer) getting on with their plan regardless of human casualties, nature being red in tooth and claw and all that. With few exceptions, the scope of Biblical evidence that "everything's going to be okay if you just have enough faith," is mighty slim.

And the context of those exceptions are evidence that exceptions are made only when they serve a pivotal historical or theological purpose. I'm highly skeptical that I meet any of that criteria in the Grand Scheme.

I studied this theology for nearly 20 years, in the Greek, and I swear – examples of saving someone from death by prayer or faith are extremely hard to come by. I think C.S. Lewis was onto something when he said, "I don't pray to change God, I pray to change me." At the very least, he realized God was not a cosmic piggy bank or genie, doling out touchdowns and cancer healings using Facebook "likes." Yes, I know – someone's brother's nieces' cousin once worked with a guy whose girlfriend was cured of warts by putting her hand on the TV with Robert Tilton and believing *really hard*. The only thing that proves is that our justice system is flawed because Tilton isn't locked away in a deep dark hole with other thieves and con-men. And that televisions are somehow deadly to warts.

There's a real problem among people of faith when it comes to the word *evidence,* too. No matter what religion they claim, they seem to not understand the difference between anecdotal evidence (personal stories) and empirical, objective evidence. But even in matters of faith, the anecdotal evidence reveals that "speaking your own health" and positive self-talk is not much more than wishful thinking. People still get sick and die, even those who believe strongly that they won't. Yes, the Bible, and other religious writings, promise "eternal glory." But in this life, they often promise suffering, pain, persecution, and death. That isn't just my take on the matter – if you subscribe to the Judeo-Christian theological framework, this is what the Bible teaches. The only way to hold the belief that "everything will work out fine" in good conscious is if you mean it in the eternal sense – as in, even if I don't survive all this, I'll go on to heaven (or paradise, or Valhalla, or wherever you plan to go). To have faith "that it will all work out" is to believe something that has never been promised to me – not by the Bible, The Universe, or anything else. I don't think anyone would disagree with that, no matter your belief system. We know it's true because we have experienced it – who among us has not lost a loved one or seen life snatched away suddenly? Even as I write this, my wife and I mourn the loss of our dear friend, Robin, who literally dropped dead at her home over the weekend. She nor anyone else had a clue that there was an infection lurking in her body, waiting for the opportune moment to strike. I'm left with no comfort in the thought that her sudden absence from our lives is for some greater good, and her husband certainly won't ever think that it all worked out for good.

When I delve into all of this, it's assumed that I'm a pessimist, or an Atheist, or that I somehow expect or even want things to end badly. Of course not. It just means that I don't and never have believed that "having faith" serves a purpose toward actual survival, because the Bible never promises physical survival (or for my non-Christian readers, the Universe, etc.). The only way to get around this fact is to cling to the aforementioned "faith/wealth" hokum. And even if you risk your mental stability trying to make it all fit into that framework your whole life long, in the end, life has a 100% mortality rate.

I don't blow off the idea of faith and hope altogether. There's significant evidence that faith and hope both help us to heal faster or even have a more positive outlook. I get that. All I can say is that believing there's a grand purpose for being sick or possibly having my life cut short brings me absolutely zero comfort. I can say with certainty that I care way more about seeing my boys get married and growing old with my wife than I do about Anyone or Anything's stupid Grand Plan or anything "working together for the good" of it. Call me selfish, but I'd rather know my grandkids, thanks. While I would never dream of telling someone *not* to have faith that things will work out well for them, promises of "things working out" have been of no comfort to me.

Here's something else I know – in my long, excruciating struggle with faith and Biblical theology, I could never digest the idea that I was unworthy of this plan, or of God because I love my father, mother, and son more than I love God (Matthew 10:37). I do love them more. I can't help it, because I'm wired to do so. It's a biological fact, proven time and again across time and cultures. It begs the question that the chamber pot is warned not to ask the potter: "Why have you made me thus?" (Romans 9:20). I will shout from the rooftops that I love my kids, wife, parents, brothers, and friends, more than I will ever be in love with a Divine Plan, or the person or deity who put it into motion, if such a thing truly exists. I'll shout as loud as I can because even though people of faith would say it's not good, at least it's true. And lying about it for the sake of appearing spiritually mature or wise only puts me in the same camp with Kenneth Hagen and Benny Hinn, who proclaim their love of God to the world, but actually love themselves, creature comforts, and money more. Plus, it's bloody exhausting. I suspect we all feel that way, deep down. I've just chosen to own up to it. This makes me a bad person in the minds of some. But at least I can look I the mirror.

If you want to put your hand on the front page of this book and send me money, I won't stop you. But I can't bank on an unseen energy to fix all my ailments. It didn't fix my HCM. It's not going to turn a plastic and rubber heart into a real one. It's not going to magically propel me to the top of the transplant waiting list. I'll get there by paying my dues, by doing my time in this room, giving up blood every day, informing my nurse about my fecal and urine volumes, and by walking my laps around this hall so my legs aren't shriveled up by the time I work my way there. I will get there by outlasting, so long as I have the capacity to do so. The time may come when I don't. So be it. I'll have done everything I needed to do. Then it will be in the hands of whatever unknown power those around me wish to ascribe it to. And hopefully, that notion will comfort them. My comfort comes from doing all of those things I listed and doing them as well as I can without complaining about it. That will be my victory, if there's one to be had.

"This," Perry said, "this right here. This is the test. Now.

Not whether or not you survive a transplant. The test is whether or not you lose yourself along the way. That's the hard part. That's the part we have control over, that we can win or lose."

Obviously, I welcome anyone's well wishes, prayers, laying on of hands, and questions of concern. But I suspect those things are more for the well-wisher than they are for me. Most of the time, I get the feeling that people are trying to convince themselves, more than trying to reassure me. This may be painful to hear, but it's something we all need to be reminded of when comforting one another. It's not the patient's job to reassure or comfort those around him/her. It's not that I don't care about the worries or anxieties of others. I really, really do. It hurts me to see the expression on the faces of friends and family as I explain what is happening here. I want to comfort them. I believe there's a give and take, and I certainly don't want to be fussed over and coddled.

Here's what I notice; many people have prayed over me, blessed me, and shared scripture with me over the last sixteen years. I don't mind this in the least, but in almost every case, I was never asked if this was something the person could do *for me*. I *love* that they care enough to do something that they think will be a comfort to me, but no one ever asks, they just assume. It's both touching and amusing because I realized long ago that they are doing this to comfort themselves. It's taught me a lot about my efforts to comfort other people in times of distress.

I derive all the comfort and assurance I need from day-to-day life. Christie, Rich, and Brennan are life affirming to me. Their zest for life and laughter give me great hope that everything will be okay. I am uplifted and comforted by music that transcends the temporal. Good food and wine have become to me a celebration of life itself. A well-told story be it in a novel, television show, movie, or game is cause for embracing life through the timeless tradition of sharing hopes, fears, and dreams through narrative. These things, at least to me, are far better, richer, and more life affirming than either assurances that it will all work out or promises of eternal rewards. I wouldn't trade watching my kids grow up for anything – temporal or eternal. I suspect most people wouldn't, if they're being honest, instead of parroting the things we all think we're supposed to say.

    All of that is enough for me. At least until I learn how to use The Force.

Chapter 15

Momentary Respite

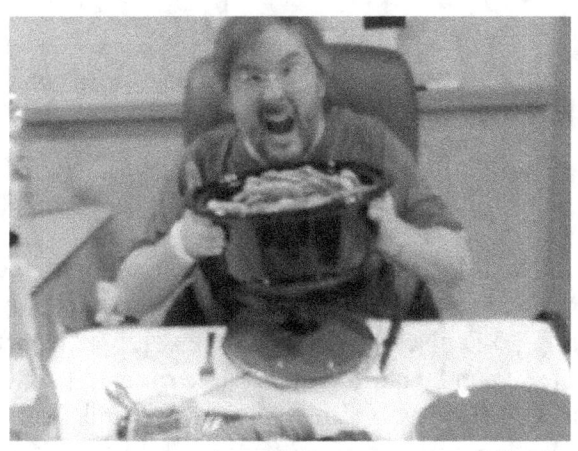

We could pretend this room is not so small
We could imagine that the window, doesn't face a brick wall
Ignore the sirens for just one night
This hour could be a momentary respite

If I could ignore the beating in my head,
And dis-remember all the things, that everybody said
Leave this place and just take flight
I'd consider it, a momentary respite

I can't see dragons and wizards in here,
Nowhere to break away, give into our fears
Can't dream of sunshine in the middle of the night
Or hope too hard for a momentary respite

If I had a way, I'd take us back in time

Conversations from Room 1170

Step from the phone booth, somewhere in 2009
I thought we'd made it through the worst part of the fight
Just for a while it was a momentary respite

I can't see spaceships or ponies in here
No time to doubt or cry, to wipe away our tears
Try to believe there's sunshine on the other side
Just a fantasy, a momentary respite

We could pretend, this room was not so small
We could imagine that life won't make dust of us all
Walk outside and lose ourselves in light
But for now, we need a momentary respite

I have a lot of downtime and sans HCM, enough energy to be productive. My goal for now is to get my music, books, and blog, all in one place online. I grab davejohnsonstuff.com and an old writer friend puts together a clearing house/website for everything. I busy myself finishing artwork and distribution for Instead of Wither and Straining Toward the Light (an album I'd recorded back in 2007 that never saw the light of day), as well as finalizing covers for my books, The Ghost of Maddingbrew and Lorenzo the Magnificent. It takes a few weeks to get it all set up on the website, which keeps my mind off of being here.

    The days slide into weeks, months. Christie brings candles and crab legs for Valentine's Day and we actually get a solid hour just to eat and talk without interruption. Her and Brennan's birthdays come and go, our twenty-fourth wedding anniversary. We've grown so used to thinking that each of these yearly events may be my last, we don't even make a big deal of it anymore. We play board games, watch Firefly, the new Star Wars movie, and eat together. Christie gets snowed in at the hospital for three days during a freak snowstorm in March and sleeps in my room during the day, woken constantly by the typical interruptions on an ICU. Our mom and daughter friends, Michelle and Dominique have essentially moved into our spare bedroom at this point and stay with the boys at night, running back to take care of their horse farm during the day.

I finally get a few bites from agents for both of my novels. Skirting the fact that I'm currently in the hospital with no heart, I send manuscripts and start discussing the possibility of representation for the books. I'm banging out revisions every day, interspersed with visits from Brian Ditzler, a post-transplant guy who's started hanging out a day or two a week. We talk music and HCM - he lost his dad and siblings, plus most of his extended family to it. Mudgeman drops by a few times a month, as do Marc and Ellen Gecker. We start a Star Wars RPG (role-playing game) with our friend Ron, and his son, Jack. Christie is forced by the hospital to enroll in school, as per her contract, and all pleas for forbearance due to our circumstance are met with well-wishes and the repeated threat of termination. She takes two easy classes and pushes through, but it only decreases the amount of rest she's getting. Other nurses catch wind of me helping her with edits and bibliographies, and I get a request for writing or editing help at least once a week from someone plugging away at their bachelors or masters. Higher education. One more thing HCM effectively robbed me of. I've started back to school so many times I can't count, but it's always interrupted by health or finances due to health. I calculate that I have the cumulative credits and experience hours to bring me just shy of a Masters, but the credits are so varied and widely dispersed between theology, Middle-Eastern history, Biblical languages, Elementary Education, media services, and sociology that they can't all be cobbled into a single degree. Educated but without papers. It's better than I'd hoped for when I was first diagnosed.

I experience the boy's lives second hand, while other people drive them to parties, the park, movies, and everything else. Of course, all of this keeps me connected to the real world, but it punctuates how everyone's life is moving forward while I'm still sitting here, waiting. Maybe for nothing. In here, time stands still.

Nurses, managers, doctors, family, and janitors come in, go out, go home, come back. They're living life in those spaces between. But I now know what Perry meant when he said, "They don't know what's going on. They just work here. I live here."

I try to stay in touch with the boys any way I can. We watch TV shows together over Skype or in the room. I spend hours building D&D maps online that we play from time to time, and keep Skype open most days to help with schoolwork when they need me. They don't, much - they've learned to be self-sufficient over the years. If anything, they're getting ahead in math and reading.

Despite all this, I can feel Rich and I growing apart. He's handled our role-reversal pretty well over the last few years, but we've had zero moments alone, just the two of us since all of this started. Brennan either. I'm beginning to realize how important those moments are. Life happens in those short moments. Rob Thomas sings, *"Life slips away, but these small hours will remain."*

Some of mine and Rich's most serious conversations have been in the car. Dealing with a younger brother, death, girls, money, the birds and the bees, religion . . . all the endpoints of meandering chit chat between Dairy Queen and home, the library and the grocery store. But we haven't had those moments in a long time. I know he's going through things. He's fifteen. Stress. Girls. Existential doubts and fears. Anxiety over his future. Things that are about him - not about me. He keeps those things to himself for the most part right now, because there's no room for them, as much as I try to clear a space. The urgency and possible finality of the everyday fills up every single empty molecule in the room, all the time. There's even less room for Brennan. Lives can't be put on hold, and theirs are going on without me, and with a mother who's trying to hold everything together and get us through this in one piece. They've become their own stability, and that means dealing with their own problems, quietly and privately. I know this is happening, and I worry there will be no way to put things back the way they should be, if I even survive this.

***

Life on the HVI is taking its toll. I spent a few blog posts trying to describe what the day to day is like.

> *My current situation is a direct result of ill-fitting and short-sighted UNOS policies. I've been implanted with an artificial heart and placed on a portable driver for the express purpose of being able to live as normal a life as possible at home with my family while awaiting transplant. Yet, because of UNOS policies, my place on the waiting list drops down into the hundreds when I go home (what's currently known as a Status 2 listing). As long as I stay admitted to the hospital, I am listed as a 1A patient, and my name rides the very top of the waiting list for O+ hearts. Due to my accumulated time here as a 1A for the last two-and-a-half years (spending two weeks at a time every 6 weeks with a swans cath on IV drugs I didn't need), my name shows up a lot when the facility gets offers – though so far, none of them have been good. So regardless of the fact that I would be safer from infection at home, as well as more closely watched and listened to (in case something goes wrong with my heart driver), here I sit, an otherwise healthy, ambulatory, independent forty-five-year-old with a family that can only be together about twice a week. The fact that I literally have no heart is irrelevant to UNOS. To their $1+1=3$ way of thinking, I'm healthy enough to live at home, therefore, my need is less urgent than someone living in the hospital. Period.*
>
> *You can imagine the abiding frustration of the situation. But living in an ICU ward as an independent, functioning, technically "non-sick" person is enough to drive anyone mad after a time.*
>
> *I'll try to put it in a context that might make more sense to the average person.*

Conversations from Room 1170

You awake in your bed to find someone drawing blood from your left arm (now, I have a permanent line they can draw from, so I don't actually get a needle every morning). This person will be your companion today. You may not even know their name yet, maybe you've never seen them before in your life. You will interact with them roughly once per hour, and they will accompany you everywhere you go. You didn't pick them. They may not even be a nice or interesting person, certainly not someone you would seek a friendship with (luckily for me, most of mine have become friends). Nevertheless, you're stuck with them for the next twelve hours, at which point they will be replaced by someone else you may or may not know. Rinse and repeat.

As you come to your senses – probably not from REM sleep because you kept waking up to the bells and noises last night – another group of four to six people enter your bedroom, a mix of acquaintances and strangers. One carries a small netbook. Another begins peppering you with questions – how are you feeling? What was your weight yesterday? Did you poop? You don't wear pajamas to sleep but try to keep yourself covered the best you can as this person squeezes your ankles and wants a detailed look at your stomach (where my drive lines are), all in view of the group. Any response you give is quickly recorded by the guy with the netbook. This is all WHILE you're still lying in bed. Before coffee. Before you've had a chance to pee. The only way around this is to put a sign on your bedroom door warning everyone not to disturb you before such-and-such o'clock, and hope they honor the request. Once they leave, your companion wheels a huge scale into your room. Don't like being in your underwear in front of strangers? Sorry – you need to step on with as little clothing as possible. You can buy your own scale for your room, but you still have to weigh on this one at least once a week. Because UNOS.

This scenario potentially happens every morning – seven days a week, but here's the catch. Those acquaintances? You never really get to know them, and you never get used to it because it's a different group of people each morning, save one or two. Good morning, sunshine!

You pee in a jug that you'll keep for your companion because they need to measure how much you produce each day. So yeah, you'll be peeing in that same jug all day, every day, and they'll record it each time. It'll start to stink eventually, and you'll have to ask for a replacement. Then you take a shower – wait no. You can't take a shower. Let's say your shower is broken indefinitely – you have to bathe and wash your hair using the sink (I haven't really showered in nine months because I can't get the PIC line in my arm, or the drive lines in my stomach, wet). This kind of works, but you still feel manky and try to deal with it using powder and lotion. You're not done yet – take your own temperature and blood pressure or let your companion do it. There are three numbers on the TAH display window that have to be recorded. You'll be doing this roughly every four hours every day, whether you're in a meeting, the middle of a meal, television show, eating a meal, having a phone conversation, enjoying a meal, trying to take a nap, or mostly while you're trying to eat a meal. Even though these numbers have been the same for four months, every single time, every four hours, for four months, you still have to do this. Because UNOS.

Time for first breakfast! A cocktail of nine pills, (most of them smell like roadkill) with water to drink. These will make you pee more, a real treat with the measuring jug (be sure to ask for hand sanitizer). Hungry yet? Yeah, you're starving. Time for second breakfast! You can have a tray delivered to your room. This morning it's scrambled liquid egg with a few canned, chopped red peppers thrown in, diced potatoes, a fruit cup (like the kind you used to eat in third grade), a cardboard carton of skim milk (because whole milk apparently kills people instantly), and some unidentifiable liquid they claim is coffee. By the way, there is no seasoning on any of this – no salt, no pepper, no butter. You receive a small packet of pepper and Mrs. Dash. The meal smells like something the Donner party wouldn't touch. Be grateful – tomorrow is turkey bacon (last used to change the oil in someone's car) and microwave pancakes. This is breakfast. Every single morning. Unless you order something different. A small box of Kellogg's cereal? Fatty sausage patties with starchy biscuits? A piece of fruit? (Be sure to check each piece for bad spots, there will be many.)

But there's hope! Since you can walk, you just go down to your kitchen and choose your own breakfast. You're starving, but your companion has to repeat your morning ritual with one to two other people who can't move around as easily – they need help getting to the bathroom, and opening the little juice cups, cutting their pancakes, etc. So, you wait. Sometimes you wait longer. Finally, your well-meaning and over-worked companion walks you down to your kitchen. You find pretty much the same options as offered on the tray. You're trying to eat as healthy as possible so if you manage to avoid the turkey bacon and greasy gravy and biscuits, you could have an omelet made from the chemical egg juice. Or maybe the yogurt. Yogurt's good for you, right? Which flavor would you like? Scooby-Doo Raspberry? Dulce de Leche with chocolate sprinkles? Ooo! How about Ghostbuster green apple! Where's the normal, healthy, unflavored yogurt, you ask? The kind for people who aren't five years old? No one knows what you're talking about. Is that a thing? There's desiccated fruit, or oatmeal. You could eat the oatmeal – that's good for you. Hope you like it A LOT because if you're going to eat healthy – it's oatmeal 7 days a week for you. Guess how quickly you'll get tired of oatmeal? I don't even want to type the word again.

You'll repeat this scenario at every meal, but also be aware that you can only eat $10 worth of food at each meal. Ever eaten anywhere but McDonald's or Taco Bell for $10? Keep in mind that whatever you choose, your companion will take note, because they are charged with your overall well-being. You do the best you can, but it's far from ideal nutrition (more on this later). You have to take the food back to your bedroom to eat (let's say for the sake of the example you live in a very large house). By the *time you get back, the food is cold. You can microwave it in a room down the hall, but some of the other people living in your house don't want you going in there – you have to get your companion to do it for you. Hopefully she doesn't get called away while you're waiting. Just obtaining breakfast in this way, even if everything goes smoothly, can take anywhere from 15 to 45 minutes front to back - that's before you start eating. Hope you're not a person who wakes up hungry, like me. It's been over an hour and a half since you were woken up. You reflect on how your life has come to a point where you can't even control when you eat your own meals.*

You finally sit down with your food, and another group enters your bedroom. I deliberately use the word "entered" because they didn't knock, they just entered. They want to ask you questions about the quality of your room, the color of the drapes, the friendliness of the acquaintances who wake you up each morning, etc. Because you're fool enough to believe that describing your morning to them will somehow make a difference in mornings to come, you actually answer their questions. They don't write any of this down, as your food gets cold once again. They thank you for your feedback, leave the room, clock out, go home, and don't remember your name or anything you said by the next day.

But they'll want to come again – maybe next week, maybe the week after. They have to do this because it's their job. But they don't actually do anything to address the problems you have. They have to keep asking the questions - it's part of what allows you to have a house in this neighborhood (in the hospital world, facilities jump through an eternity of hoops to maintain what is called "magnet status" - an honor that looks good on the banner out front, but is only achieved by meaningless protocols inflicted on the nursing staff, lots of circle-jerk committees that are little more than a waste of time, and lots and lots of student debt from pushing floor nurses to get a Master degree so they can be part of the management that creates the aforementioned protocols and committees (note that this run on sentence doesn't include the phrase "patient care" even once). You're just a tool to help them keep up the status of the house, the neighborhood - though you'll never personally benefit from these questions.

You can (as I have) put another sign on the door informing all visitors that they need permission from your companion before they can enter your room. You quickly become astounded at the illiteracy rate of the people living in your house. Now – make sure that each day, you point this sign out to your companion (because it may be a new person every day) so they will keep these intrusions to a minimum. But remember there will be times in the privacy of your bedroom when you're changing clothes, peeing in your jug, having a private or intense conversation with a loved one (you may die tomorrow, by the way, so understand my full-meaning when I use the adjective "intense"), or just having a good cry. If your companion is away helping one of their other charges, not watching your room, people will just (to be continued tomorrow)

I cut the blog post off abruptly here because I'm actually interrupted by someone throwing open my door without knocking. I pick it up in the next post on the following day, right where I left off:

walk right in without knocking.

Believe it or not, the writing of yesterday's post was interrupted in EXACTLY the way I was describing at that very moment. The new Chaplain came in WHILE I was typing that last sentence. No knock, no invitation. So, I couldn't finish my thought. I CAN NEVER FINISH MY THOUGHT.

As, I was saying – if the nurse isn't watching, people just…come in. Now, you can be a jerk and yell at them and tell them to get out. But it's not like shooing a salesman off your porch.

You're going to see this guy in the halls about three times a week as long as you live in this house. Do you really want to yell and be a jerk to everyone who barges into the room? Maybe you should, but there are social repercussions. It doesn't take long to develop a reputation as being grumpy, ill-tempered, "stressed out," or "that guy with all the signs on his door." So, you have to just deal with it, sorry. Make sure you wear clean underwear because you literally don't ever know who's going to see you in them. Or see them around your ankles.

The worst of these types of incidents are what I call the "finger people." Imagine that while you're sitting in your room, you're waiting on something. In my case a heart. But maybe for you, it's the callback for your dream job, or the phone call confirming your pregnancy. Maybe a loved one has been missing and you're waiting to hear from the police. Or the answer to a marriage proposal. Fill in the blank with the thing that would stress you out the most – how about the call to tell you whether or not the cancer was benign? Except you won't get this news by phone. It will be delivered personally to your room, probably by someone you don't know and have never met. So, you're in a constant state of anticipation. For months.

Without a knock, the door swings open. There stands someone you don't recognize, and they seem very hurried and excited. Is this it? Is this the moment you've been waiting for? Could it finally be happening? The wait has been agonizing (in my case, four years), but maybe today is the day. All these thoughts flash through your mind as the person holds up a wait-a-second finger so they can hear someone talking to them further down the hall.

You know the 'wait a second finger,' right? Remember when you tried to interrupt your mom while she was talking, and she'd hold up her index finger toward you without looking at you? That one. This person is talking hurriedly to someone, but you only hear her side of the conversation. Is it about that Big Thing you've been waiting for?

She walks away, but leaves the door open, because she's coming back. Of course, she's coming back. They have big news to tell you and it's urgent, so she's just left the door open for a second while they make sure they have the details of your Big News right. You continue to stare at the doorway, imagining all the phone calls you need to make to share your Big Moment with those closest to you, so they in turn can pass it on to all those who have been waiting with you, hoping and praying for you for so long, that you'll get the News you want, that you need, in order to get on with your life.

And you wait.

And you wait.

5 minutes. The suspense is killing you.

10 minutes. You can't take it anymore.

You step into the hall to find . . .

(Hang on a minute. A new cleaning guy just stopped in to clean your room, and even though you're hanging by your toenails waiting for this Person to come back – or maybe you're just trying to read a blog post and the author keeps interrupting himself – the cleaning person insists on making small talk about the weather, your (now cold) food, the television show they watched last night, or whatever. This goes on for about five minutes)

So, you step into the hall and the person isn't there. You ask around and find out that no, they really didn't need you for anything, they just had the wrong room. (This has happened to me three

Hang on – nurse is here to get vitals again.

times now with the X-Ray team). You sit back down, try to eat your cold food, and you keep waiting. And waiting.

I hate finger people. I want to break their finger.

Time for lunch – wait for your companion, then off to the kitchen again. Remember to eat healthy!

Today's choices:

Cheese steak with what looks like Oscar Meyer beef slices, canned Nacho cheese, raw onions, and a cold hoagie bun.

Buttermilk Fried Chicken, greasy "creole" cabbage (there is no seasoning on this cabbage and adding a rich adjective doesn't make it so. It's unseasoned, steamed cabbage), BLT pasta salad – Oo! Look at all that bacon!

Ground "Beef" BBQ (actual beef doesn't smell like toe jam. What is this stuff?), with baked beans, and cold (well, warm) slaw (you're allergic to mayo, so no slaw for you. Pick another veggie).

Curry (curry sauce from a can, enough salt to kill an entire continent) with fatty chicken, overcooked shrimp, or flavorless basmati rice (the people behind the counter couldn't pick ginger out of a spice line-up, even if you made them snort it).

Sushi! A healthy alternative! And it actually looks good! But you can't get that – you're not allowed to use your $10 meal ticket on the sushi. You actually thought they were going to make healthy food available to eat? Joke's on you. Move along. That's only for the people visiting the house.

Pizza, slathered in greasy pepperoni or sausage, and high-salt mozzarella cheese. You'll need a pair of tongs to retrieve a slice from the grease pond it's floating in.

Hey look! There's a whole counter with healthy choices like couscous, low-carb pasta salads, and veggie mixes. You can get something from there or buy a drink to go with your meal. But you can't do both. Upon closer inspection, the sodium content of most of these is at least 580 mg per serving. Same for both of today's soups.

How about a sandwich? Which fatty, sodium laden, Oscar Meyer lunchmeat would you like on it? Or a salad – wait, you can't eat a lot of green leafy veggies because it affects your blood coagulation too much and could do harm. Skip the salad.

Don't even think about trying to get a full meal, a drink, and a piece of fruit or a cookie for your $10 voucher, or you'll have to go out of pocket every meal.

Get a drink – would you like a soda, a chemically enhanced diet soda, skim milk, or sugary fruit juice? Or there's weird stuff like Basil flavored Coconut Water, or lab-created "energy" drinks (I tried one of these a few weeks ago and nearly re-enacted the chest bursting scene from Alien, except with my intestinal tract; avoid). You can drink water, of course. For every meal. Three times a day. For months on end. They also have milkshakes. But watch your blood sugar level!

Okay, did you pick something? Great! Follow your companion back to your room. Your food is cold again so hopefully you didn't get anything that won't microwave.

Or maybe you didn't pick anything. Maybe your spouse brought up some food to your small refrigerator in the other bedroom. Or maybe you yourself made something and put it there. It's way healthier and tastier than anything in your kitchen, and you made enough to last for the week, for situations just like this.

You go to retrieve that food. But alas, it's not there. The food policeman who lives in your house with you threw it away. Why? Because it was more than three days old. Didn't you know that all food, no matter what it is, spoils after three days? You didn't need the containers the food was in did you? Hope not, because they're gone too. Maybe you should have just gotten the fried chicken.

Screw it – you call Domino's or the Chinese place from your room and have it delivered. By this time, your stomach has started eating itself. The food arrives. It's hot, it's fresh, it's full of preservatives and sodium, but no more so than the food in your kitchen you decided not to eat.

You lift a bite to your mouth.

The door opens. It's a dietitian. An illiterate dietitian. She slipped past your companion, just like the Chaplain. The staff has been so kind as to ask them to come talk to you about your food choices. She informs you that at each meal, you should try to eat:

1) A card-deck sized portion of lean meat (I'm assuming in this case that would be the overcooked shrimp from the curry that you didn't get because you don't even like Indian food – unless that "beef" was actually hedgehog or mongoose, in which case you should have went with the BBQ. At least I think hedgehog and mongoose are considered "lean").

2) A vegetable – did you pick the flavorless cabbage (assuming you like cabbage), one of the many starches posing as veggies, the mayo-based coleslaw from a can? No? Well, you could just eat a salad, she says. The ones you really need to avoid because you'll die? Yeah. Those salads.

3) A starch – those are plentiful, in fact they comprise about 75% of the food in your kitchen. You never realized there were four-hundred and fourty-six ways to prepare a potato, but someone in your kitchen does!

After a quasi-scolding about your food choices, you choke down your cold pizza. Wait – where are you going? Uh-uh. You're staying in your room all day. You *might* be able to get your companion to take you to another room or even outside later, but it's raining outside. It's always raining. It's like living in Seattle or London. But crappier.

Next: you're going to try to write an e-mail, or a heartfelt letter to a loved one, or watch a fourty-four-minute television episode. This will require a few uninterrupted thoughts and a bit of concentration. Brace yourself.

And the final blog post on day three:

You've not been out of your house for nearly four months now, but you're keeping it together because you have a project to work on. For me, it's the revision of an 84,000-word novel. Maybe you're putting together your resume for that dream job. Or interviewing for it over the phone. Or maybe you just want some privacy to think, pray, meditate, or finish whatever project you're working on. It could be any of those things – we all know how it is to be interrupted when we're "in the zone." These are just some examples to think of. But for the sake of simplicity, let's say instead of taking your sink bath this morning, you decided to do it after lunch.

So, you're exiting your bathroom, as clean as it's possible to get in the sink and headed for your small closet (that's just next to the bedroom door). There's a quick knock and the door flies open. There stands a younger person of the opposite sex – a total stranger – and you're wearing nothing but a surprised look. They hurriedly apologize and close the door, but they're outside, waiting for you to get dressed. You scramble to get dried off and clothed as quickly as possible because you know from experience that while it takes the average person about one to two minutes to do this, the person outside your door isn't counting down those two minutes in real time. They're going to knock on the door about every 15-20 seconds until you're dressed, and there's no guarantee that they won't throw open the door a second time without your consent (if you're connected to a TAH, getting dressed takes longer than normal because you're working around the cannula sites in your abdomen and trying to wrap an abdominal binder under your shirt). After frantically getting dressed, and mostly still wet, you open the door. This person is there to scan the "equipment" in your room.

Oh, by the way, they're scanning your furniture, so they can charge you for it – approximately $2500 per day for using your bedroom, the bed, the chair, and your bathroom. This is the part I wish I was just making up – because you've been here for 93 days for grand total of $232,500. Add $2500 per day that you'll be there until you incur the balloon payment – in my case for transplant – at the end where you can tack on another $997,000 – also not a made-up number - and that's only if something unexpected doesn't happen that will add to that cost. So as of today, you're in the hole $1,229,500. This might be a good time to whip out a calculator to see what percentage of that will be a co-pay. Keep a tissue box nearby – because while you've been incurring this bill, your family is living on your spouse's paycheck (which is enough to support approximately 2.5 people) and a small percentage of whatever you claimed on your tax return in 1997. You are not currently able to earn additional income because you're trapped in your bedroom. You start to warm to the idea of a universal health care system and the public hangings of medical insurance CEO's. Also, Walter White from Breaking Bad doesn't seem so crazy anymore…

So, your new friend scans the furniture and you settle back into what you were doing. Peace at last. You can finally focus on th-

DING - BONG

DING - BONG

DING - BONG

DIT DIT DIT……DIT DUU

DIT DIT DIT……DIT DUU

BLAT!!! BLAT!!! BLAT!!!!

You've almost learned to ignore all the sounds coming from the other rooms, but sometimes they go on and on and on and on and on and on and on and on and on and %^*&%@# on until you want to murder kittens with your bare hands. Put headphones on? Gotta be careful about that because if the TAH alarms go off for some reason, you won't hear them. Just try harder to focus. Focusing... focusing... focusing... Time for your meds and vitals again! How much work did you get done?

You give up and decide to go for a walk. You're not allowed to go anywhere but the bedroom and hallway, but you need at least some exercise, so you pace the circular hallway. Around and around and around. Every person you pass asks how you're doing. You want to refer them to these blog posts. You mumble an acknowledgment and keep pacing. A new group enters the hall – a mix of acquaintances and strangers. They're attending to people in the other rooms. The crazy thing about this group is that when they appear, you disappear. They stand in bunches in the middle of the hall, forcing you to walk around or through them. As they move from room to room, they clip your shoulder or elbows in their hurry. The scariest thing about this is that you're wearing a backpack with tubes coming out of the side, and they're connected to your abdomen by stitches and a very tight bandage. But they stick out a little bit, meaning you need wider clearance than the average person. You're very worried that these tubes will get caught on something or someone, so crowded places are not your friend. But this new group doesn't seem to notice the tubes connecting the backpack to your artificial heart – the very thing keeping you alive from moment to moment. They brush against them, they bump into them, without any acknowledgement of your existence. Eventually, you give up trying to walk because it feels too dangerous and you go back to your room. You've been asking the People In Charge for about a month for a treadmill or exercise bike so you can exercise in a safer way – you've even seen both pieces of equipment – they're at the end of the hall, not being used by anyone. But the weeks roll by and when you continually ask, you're told about paperwork, schedules, authorizations, and protocols that are beyond your scope of understanding, but are meant to serve as an excuse for lack of progress with the treadmill or bike. So, you sit in a chair, feeling your strength ebb away and your muscles weaken each day. You've been told over and over that you'll recover from this confinement (and surgery, in my case) more quickly and successfully the more fit you are going into the procedure. Despite this, there is little to no effort made to help you stay fit – just the jostling monotony of trying to walk in the hall, fearful that you're going to get hurt, or possibly die.

You run your tongue over your teeth. It feels disgusting, despite regular brushing. You're overdue for a teeth cleaning. You can go downstairs to get your teeth cleaned (after asking the People In Charge for three months), but you'll have to a) be put under anesthesia, b) get disconnected from the portable heart pump and connected to a large machine on wheels because "it's protocol" (it will generally take about 3-4 days to be put back on the backpack, meaning you're largely confined to the chair or bed in your room for that period of time). You're also not supposed to eat until after the cleaning tomorrow, despite the fact that the only reason you wouldn't eat is if you're going under anesthesia – which I'm pretty sure no one does when having their teeth cleaned. What time will it be? Take a wild guess! You could go without food from midnight tonight until 8pm tomorrow. Hopefully it will be in the morning, but there's no way to know. Why do you have to fast before a teeth cleaning? Because "it's protocol." There's no medical necessity for it. It's just The Way Things Are Done and asking for an exception based on common sense is met with confusion and impatience. Why are you holding up the process?

You give up on getting your teeth cleaned – despite being told by The People In Charge that it's important to go into your upcoming surgery with optimal dental health because the mouth is the #1 source of infection and can cause the whole thing to fail, resulting in (worst case scenario, death) all kinds of problems.

You give up on exercise. You give up on having a place to keep your food without it being randomly thrown away. It's rained so much, you give up on believing you'll ever see the sun again or feel a breeze on your face. You'd be happy to go outside in the rain, but you can't get your backpack pump wet. And it's cold. Best you can do is sit and stare out the window at the brick wall of an adjacent building.

It's time for bed. Have you recorded everything you've drank and all your urine for the day? Did you check your vital signs all five times? Leave any food in the fridge that may get thrown away? You like to read before you go to bed but despite repeated requests for the dead lightbulb over the bed to be changed, it still hasn't been. Getting into and out of bed is a real production so you set things up where you don't have to. TAH pump on the table at bedside, along with a water bottle and urinal. You'll need to put the urinal in the bed with you each time you pee (hope you're a good aim). The bed mattress is covered in vinyl – easy to clean. but it doesn't breathe, so you wake up each night four or five times in a pool of your own sweat and shift around to find a dry spot. Sometimes you can't. You're lying on your back the entire night because to lay on your side causes pain at your cannula site. The sweat is the worst because you can't shower, so you do your best to get the stink off every morning and ask your companion to change the bed sheets.

Sleep is the only escape from all of it and you finally, restlessly drift off...

GET THE HELL OUT OF HERE! I'M GONNA KICK YOUR ASS!!!!

Just ignore that – it's the delirious elderly woman in the next room threatening the nurses at the top of her lungs. She'll scream a variety of threats and vulgar insults throughout the rest of the night and into the morning hours. Sometimes they wake you up, but eventually you're too exhausted and just sleep through them. It goes on most of the next day while you're trying to rest, work, or have a serious conversation with one of your kids, or your spouse who you've not seen in three days.

Don't worry, she'll fade into the call bells, bustle, fire drill alarms, bed alarms, and code alarms. Your room is across from the meeting place of the People In Charge, who are for the most part quiet and respectful during the night. But from time to time, one of the companions, or someone from elsewhere in the house stands in the hall between the two rooms and has loud conversations filled with laughter and exclamations. You finally fall asleep wondering how many more days this will go on. For some people, these are the last experiences they'll ever have. You hope that's not how it turns out for you, but there are no assurances. There's just the intrusions, the frustrations, the isolation, the measuring, the labs, the sweating, and most of all, the waiting.

* * *

I think about Perry a lot. He lived in this very room for months before his transplant. He had migraines and couldn't get an eye exam. He had back pain from the bed, so slept in the chair. He was nineteen years old. Nineteen. He never got to see a dream fulfilled, or even fail really. He never dated or had sex. He never knew the joy of holding his own child, or even a niece or nephew. He never got to travel much and hadn't even tried Indian food until I forced it on him.

He didn't complain. He didn't rage against the TAH or predicament. He just did what had to be done and he didn't truck with other people feeling sorry for him because he had to do it. He understood frailty, fear, and weakness. But he didn't use those as a shield to hide behind or as a sword to lash out at other people.

I lapse into self-pity at times. I do. But then there's Perry, in my head, like some kind of prankster Obi-Wan-Kenobi, saying, "Quit whining. You have to do this, so just do it. Also slip some laxative into Josh's coffee if you get a chance." That was pretty much the core of his uncomplicated philosophy about pain and suffering. So, I have no excuse for whining.

I find myself slipping more and more into a dreamlike state, where I stare out the window at the brick wall until my eyes go glassy. I dig deep into my memory and try to pull out every little detail of life in Bentonville, what now feels like a lifetime ago. Sitting in the library, drinking tea and watching the leaves fall. Watching the kids play with their friends at the park, while in the company of my own friends. Basking in the normalcy and security of it all. I can feel Brennan's hand in mine as we make our way into the gym, or the library for Storytime. I can see Rich and I in our Watchdog Dad t-shirts, sitting together with his classmates at lunch in the cafeteria of the school we loved so much. Feel the sidewalk under my feet and hear the electric motor of the boy's riding truck, Christie and I following behind with Nanouq as we walked around the block after dinner each night. It's a moment I've captured perfectly in my mind, and I go there to escape from this place, this time, this...thing that our lives have become. I know I shouldn't, because it only makes things worse. It's something I can never get back and dwelling on it just makes this all that much harder. But I'm becoming addicted to it - living in that place in my mind. I wonder if this is how people develop delirium and dementia. When life has turned sour and they can't cope with their present reality, they just turn their mind back to a better place and time, like switching channels on a television. Maybe they start out doing it as a momentary respite, a small reward to themselves for getting through another day. And it's so peaceful there, they linger just a bit longer, going more often. Until finally, they decide it's better there, in that place that Once Was, and they should just stay, willingly trapped there, and present reality becomes nothing more than a dream state, something they wake up from into their perfect world.

It's like a drug. I'm starting not to be able to imagine much of anything anymore - not melodies for songs, not ideas for new books or stories. TV no longer holds my interest. I just want to go back to the way things were, even if only for a few minutes. No matter what happens, even in the best-case scenario, I don't think I'll ever have that much peace and contentment again. So I can only have it in my fantasy, and I go there every night when I'm falling asleep, and I go there again when I wake up in the morning. I go there when my mind drifts from trying to watch TV, and even in the middle of playing a video game. It's the only place I can go to get away from this horror movie, and maybe one day, I'll go there and not come back. I doubt I'll even know that my reality has flipped, then I'm thinking backwards and dreaming while wide awake. At least there, I can be with Christie, and Rich, and Brennan, and Nanouq all the time. Here, I'm by myself, no matter who visits, no matter how many times people insert themselves into my presence every day. I try not to be, but I think I'm slipping.

Jamie's gone now too, beyond my reach. I'm the only TAH patient left in the building. They finally got the pediatric TAH to maintain a steady pressure, so she shipped out to Philly, despite Dr. Brehm's raging protestations. They won't transplant her here. After losing both Jo and Perry, it's too much of a risk to the program. She's ill, malnourished and atrophied from being in a bed for a year and a half. I wonder if I'll see her again - she'll live in Philly when this is all over. Our brotherhood has broken up and we're beyond helping each other now. I don't know that we have anything left to give each other anyway.

Chapter 16

Village

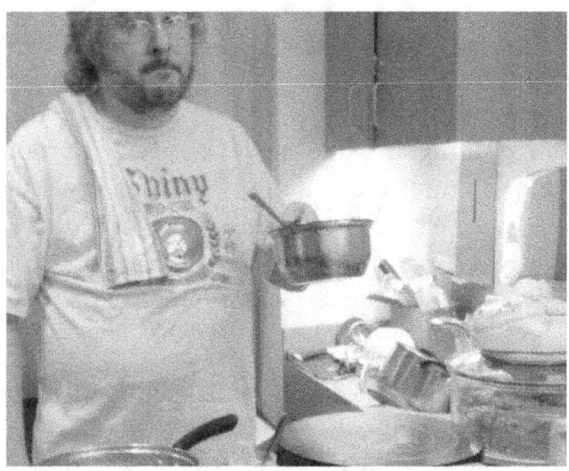

Butchers, bakers, candlestick makers
Doctors, lawyers, Indian chiefs
Janitors in face masks, X-ray, device techs
Gowns and machines swirling all around me

It takes a village, you'd best believe
You'll know it if you ever spend a year down on your knees
It takes a village, you know it's true
Tell me from six feet down, what you'd rather do
(just settle in)

Nurses writing papers, nursing every hangnail
Shift change, dawn of the dead
Needle jocks, baby docs, residents in deadlock

Conversations from Room 1170

Shirts, ties, and shrinks, all to help me clear my head

Hanging out in dry dock, living for the punch clock
Who'll creep with me tonight?
Musician and liaison, coordination payoff
Engineers, scalpel jocks, get me to the next fight

I've developed a sense of ownership.

When you live on a hospital unit, you watch other people's lives swirling around you, while your life stands still (other than the occasional stroke or fluid restriction change). You're the one walking around at night, while nurses are busy in rooms and the doctors, therapists, managers, and visitors are gone. You start to feel like you own the place, not in the sense that you run it, but in the sense that everyone else only sees part of the picture, while you get to stand back and observe the culture, the ebb and flow. Like Perry said, they just work here. I live here.

I know that JACO is doing an inspection this week. They'll show up unannounced, and the unit has to pass safety and cleaning inspections, so I'm clearing the soda cans and dry foods out of my window sill, stashing them in my personal bins and boxes, which they can't look in. I hide my cookware away and even disconnect my XBox from the room monitor. I shouldn't care; the nurses should be making me do all of this, but there's that sense of ownership. This place has become my home, and as odd as it may sound, I want it to succeed. The nurses work hard, and deal with death on a daily basis. Not to mention, they've been empathetic enough to let me bend the rules so that I don't lose my mind in here. I don't want JACO busting them because I'm cluttering up the sink with my dishes (begging the question, "why does the patient need his own dishes?").

It's a form of Stockholm Syndrome. I'm not being held against my will, but I am staying here unwillingly. I've always tried to be as comfortable as possible no matter what situation I'm in. It's one of the best traits you develop as a military kid, moving around, changing schools and houses, living in temporary quarters at times, and not really having a lot of control over what's going to happen next. That may sound terrible to some people, but I consider it an invaluable life skill that I wouldn't have learned otherwise. Now, when faced with the risk of the unknown, Christie, the boys, and I typically shrug and say, "we can do anything for three months!" Because we have. The trick is to loosen your grip on possessions and creature comforts. When you consider that our ancestors used to eat raw meat and bathe in the rain, going without Netflix or a smartphone for a while isn't all that tough. I've learned that I need a lot less than I have.

So that's what's happened. My world is this room for now. I have my guitar, my laptop to write with, and short that, paper and pencil. I've fixed my food situation to be tolerable, and the XBox is the icing on the cake. My friend, Hugh Hollowell (Mindi's husband) is a Mennonite minister who served the homeless community in Raleigh, North Carolina, and he says, "When you cross paths with ugliness and sorrow on a daily basis, it's imperative that you surround yourself with beauty and things that make you happy." Something like that. Accordingly, I keep my acoustic guitar at arm's length, a Terry Pratchett novel by my bed, and shortcuts to The Beatles and King's X playlists on my phone and laptop. I've changed my screen saver to rotate pictures of our family during happier times and keep my white board filled with cartoons and Douglas Adams quotes.

Beyond the room, I use the patient food room a lot; the sink, the fridge, the supplies. So, I end up in there about once a week, cleaning the fridge, sink, and microwave, organizing and restocking the little cans of juice and sodas, the silverware, peanut butter, and crackers. Night shift never washes their coffee mugs or the crock pot when they use it, so I've taken that on as my job too.

These people have become my tribe, too. I know what days Larry is off, and that Chuck will be cleaning my room those days.

I know what's going on with their kids, we talk music, and Larry talks sports, if nothing else just to help me carry on a conversation with other people. No matter which nurse I have that day, Larry and Chuck are mainstays. They laugh when I say it, but I think they have the most important job in the place. I'm at high risk for infection, and if the unit isn't clean, I could be in serious trouble. When I come back from transplant, I'll be in a new room, at an even more heightened risk for contagions and infections. But one of them will have cleaned the place and they'll do a better job than I would do myself (and I used to own a cleaning company!)

I know what's going on with Cassie's boyfriend's natural tea business. Krista's handicapped husband and grandmother. Mark's car search and Erica's kids. With all the nurses steadily taking some class or other, I end up doing some shotgun tutoring in grammar and sentence structure. The stories go on and on, but the short of it is, I'm a resident here, and it's hard not to feel like I work here too. I'm very low maintenance because I'm just sitting around waiting for a heart. But I know that once that coin flips I'll probably be the most demanding patient they've ever had, deprived of what little independence I have now, and very picky about the way things are done. I'm storing up goodwill. They find it funny.

Beyond the HVIC, I end up on Christie's unit many of the nights she works. I'm thick as thieves with Priscilla and Francis, two nurses from Kenya who pray for me constantly and always make me feel like I'm the most important person in the world, even amid the whirlwind of the trauma overflow unit. The entire crew up there thinks Christie and I are "just the cutest couple." It's a much-needed change of scenery from the HVI, and they've all become part of my tribe.

Back in my room, I can expect Greg, the chaplain to drop by about once a week. He doesn't do much "chaplaining" with me anymore.

"You're an odd duck, theologically speaking," he told me once. "I've never met a Calvinist who believes in free will."

"If I believe in either," I said. "I'm a product of the Calvary Chapel movement, Rez Band, Rich Mullins, and really liberal fist century Pharisaic doctrine."

"Yeah. I don't know what to do with that," he laughs.

Now we talk about the nature of belief in general, but mostly we talk about Brennan Manning and Chesterton, and the things we wish would change on the HVI to better serve the families of long-term care patients.

The Wizard empties my sharps bin every Tuesday, stopping in his harried schedule for only a minute or so to answer questions about Dungeons and Dragons 2.0, since the boys and I have started playing over the Roll20 web service now. He's a walking encyclopedia and we share a mutual awe of Gary Gygax (the originator of D&D). I never learn his name – he's just "the Wizard" - but he becomes part of my tribe.

The truth is, all of this will pass. This place is a job for all of these people, and they'll eventually move on from it, just as I will, like all patients do, either out the door with their family or to the morgue in a bag. I struggle mightily with these changes on the other side of transplant, but at this moment in time, for these months, the only way I can cope with the experience is to fancy myself a caretaker of sorts. The notion is, of course, ridiculous, but it gives me a much-needed sense of community, cut off from friends and any hope of maintaining a consistent social life on the outside. No one ever dis-abuses me of this illusory construct. They just eat the food I make, hang out near my door or across the hall and watch movies with me on the big monitor that I'm not supposed to use, bring me their papers to proofread, and ask how my (Medici) book is coming along. What am I listening to today? What am I reading? When are the boys coming in? What new game are we going to play? I'd like to think it's because they really care, but I suspect they're just very good at what they do and trying to get me through this whole thing alive with my sanity intact.

The circle grows each week. The human services staff. The cafeteria employees. Travel nurses just passing through. The only people held outside of my tribe are the residents. They're docs in training. They irritate and condescend to the nurses in large part, which wins them zero points with me. When I walk my laps around the unit during the weekdays, they don't move out of the way. They're "doctors," you see. Burgeoning legends in the history of medical care; I wouldn't trust them with a band-aid and a tube of Neosporin. If I passed in front of them grabbing my chest, the best of them would pee themselves and scream for the nearest nurse. I love the look on their faces when their attending stops me somewhere in their second week and asks about the family, proceeding to carry on a ten-minute conversation about the new Star Wars movie, the book they're reading, asking me if I've heard of such-and-such band. All while they stand there and wait. They see their attending docs as god-like, not to be chatted with about science fiction and Greta Van Fleet's new song. The attendings do it on purpose, to bring them down a notch, and I don't mind a bit being part of that process. And God help any of them that throw open the door to my room at 5 a.m. They learn quick that even a guy with an artificial heart can chuck a full urinal across a room with decent aim. Perry used to lose his mind with them too, and for the same reason. Nothing with me changes much from one day to the next, and I came to an agreement with the docs early on to be exempted from assessments every morning at five a.m. I will cut someone.

But my tribe, they get it. They know that it's going to take everyone to get me through this. Any transplant patient. They contend with Jamie's malaise and unwillingness to eat and my fits of rage when my food gets tossed from the patient fridge. They get that I need my space. This is my home for now. Most defend my privacy vigilantly, especially Big Mark and Chips (Justin) my usual day nurses. There are always "quality assurance," skin assessment people, and various suit and tie types trying to justify their paycheck with some nonsense about patient care, that pull rank and muscle past him, despite his warnings that they're about to meddle in the affairs of dragons. I wonder if they ever notice the "I told you so" grin on Big Mark's face as they exit the room abruptly. I'm not mean. In fact, I'm very polite to these people. Direct, but very, very polite. To the point that it's creepy. I could drop dead at any moment, and they are not part of my tribe. They are part of the mechanism that creates more stress and anxiety for patients, families, and my nurses than anything else. I am the dragon. They are crunchy and taste good with ketchup.

I come to understand why Perry was so demanding about his privacy, and why he was so judicious about who he allowed or banned from his circle. You just don't care what people think anymore, and breath is too precious to waste on poll taking or doing random analysis of the nursing staff's performance.

It really is a form of Stockholm Syndrome. You don't want to be in this place. The smell of it permeates everything. Your clothes, your hair. When you go to sleep at night you know that you smell like it too. But this is how we cope. We surround ourselves with as much beauty as we can. We try to make a space for ourselves in the world, no matter how temporary, tenuous, or cramped.

In 2004, I wrote a song called Straining Toward the Light which became the title track of that album, eventually released in 2016 alongside Instead of Wither. When my soul-sister from Calvary Chapel, Leslie, moved to Illinois for school around that time, mine and Christie's hearts were broken. It was a smart move on her part, but it left a gaping hole in our lives that no one else has ever been able to fill. We'd finished packing her and Jason's - her husband at the time - apartment, but there was some type of huge potted plant that they couldn't take and didn't want to throw away. I lugged it back to my office at home, where it sat at the end of my desk. I hated the thing because it reminded me of that day when we had to say goodbye and they were gone, beyond my reach. I'm terrible with plants, and this thing suffered unconscionable neglect. After a few months, there was nothing left but a withering trunk that twisted a foot or two above its pot. As I looked more closely one day, I realized that the trunk had actually begun bending as it died - toward the window overlooking the front yard. The only source of natural light in the room. One tiny leaf held on for dear life at the tip end. Straining Toward the Light. The lyrics popped into my head instantly:

> *When darkest shadow kills the last green thing –*
> *it spirals aimlessly away*
> *When all that used to keep you watered and warm*
> *withers down to decay*
> *All of our groaning, all our searching in the sky*
> *All of our chasing after everything that dies*
> *All our praying, and all our getting high*
> *Is so much straining - straining toward the light*
> *We're all just straining - straining toward the light*

(Straining Toward the Light – Dave Johnson)

I never pull the shutters down in my room, like Perry did. He wanted darkness to better see the TV screen, but artificial light has a depressing effect on me. I wanted as much sunlight in the room as possible, regardless of what maintenance worker could peer in on their way to the punch-clock via the alley between my room and the adjacent building. Sunlight is a piece of the outside world, a thing of beauty that I can let in every day. Anyone with hope strains toward whatever light they can find. For me, it's the sun, it's my family, but it's very much my tribe, these people to whom I've become a fixture, just part of the landscape of their workplace. They don't treat me like it, but they're used to me being here now, just like they got used to Perry. And I'm used to them. I'm invested in their struggles, their stories, their lives. This should never happen between patients and staff, but we are light to one another, and it's inevitable. To a lesser extent than my family, they've seen me through these last battles - the years of swans caths and extended stays. The A-fib and cardioversions. The TAH surgery and recovery. Dot's death. Perry's death. We all know that it will take all of us, even Larry the cleaning guy, to get me to transplant, and beyond. They're not exactly in the trenches with me, but they're frantically dropping ammo and rations from above. And so, we become war buddies, and this place that I don't want to be is both home and battlefield. It's where I may spend the last days of my life, where my family may have their final memories of me. So, I both cherish it and hate it in a way I can't quite understand. If I knew how difficult it would be to let go of if later, I may have held myself back from taking ownership, from investing. Probably not. But there are times I wish I could go back and do it differently. My lack of caution about this comes back to bite me later.

Chapter 17

Requiem for a Savior

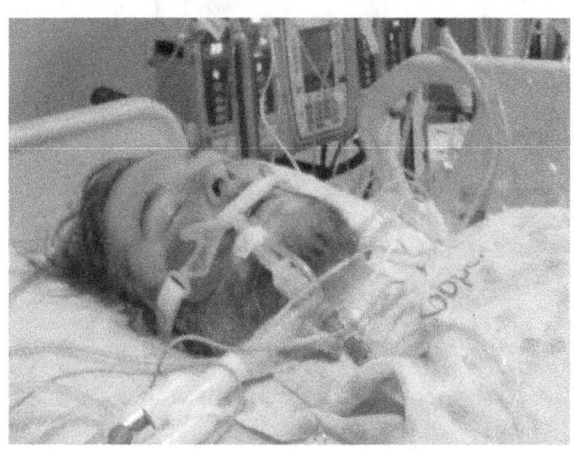

Soak it up now, it may not be too long,
Fate & circumstance conspire to make us one
Be all you are, find what is true…
and peace to you, peace to you

Where are you tonight?
I'm still wondering, I'm still crumbling
If the timing is right, it might be,
the beginning and end of something beautiful
I don't know what fate the days hold for you
I number mine like precious jewels
A beautiful tragedy, that somehow our paths will meet,
And you will come find me

I don't know who you are, but I know,

Conversations from Room 1170

I wouldn't be me without you
Is your heart enough like mine
that they might intertwine forever?
They think you're silent now, but you sins inside me

How are you tonight?
I'm still breathing, I'm still grieving
If the stars align, it might give our lives
just a little more meaning
The moment the light left your eyes,
it lit up the darkness in mine
A terrible mystery tangled in joy and misery,
That we will never meet

I don't believe time heals all pain,
So I'll carry yours and mine and probably all the blame
And number every single tear, bathed in light and bitterness here
Where hope and sorrow are alive, just like me,
just like you will always be

"It is live? Oh, I hope it's live!"

Christie is escorting me down to Starbucks in the lobby for breakfast and I hear a familiar sound floating up the corridor toward us. It's been a horrible morning – new nurse, messed up blood draw that had to be repeated, and the Freedom Driver is making a funny squeaking sound that no one can identify. We've just had another argument with Dr. Brehm about changing out my PICC line. It's still clean but they change it by protocol every three months and I'm overdue. There's been a lot of confusion and mis-read orders resulting in me getting the line replaced, only to learn it also needed to be moved to the other arm. We're furious and he's frustrated. We call a cease-fire to get coffee.

I've heard this sound for years – on Peter Gabriel, Kip Winger, Sting, and Yes albums, but always buried in the mix, uncredited, unacknowledged…it makes me crazy. Some type of melodic percussive instrument, not a steel drum, something subtler, like a subdued hand bell chorus. The hospital has instrumental music in the foyer a few times a week. It's got to be live.

We turn the corner to Starbucks to see a woman seated on a low stool, tapping out a rhythmic pattern on what looks like a small, bronze flying saucer with about eight half-dollar sized indentions around the perimeter. I'm mesmerized – it's one of the most melancholy, dark, and yet joyous sounds I've ever heard. Christie steps into the line to get coffee while I stand and stare. She notices my interest and waves me over.

"What is it called?" I sound like I'm begging her to tell me. It's been maddening to love an instrument so much and have no idea what it's called or even what it looks like.

"It's a hang (spelled "hung")," she says, "want to give it a try?"

I have no idea how to play it but considering the Freedom Driver might give a final squeak and shut off without warning, why not seize the moment?

It's like playing a piano but there's no fear of hitting the wrong key. She explains that there are a variety of sizes, all tuned to a single key – hers is in C. It's a drummer's dream.

"I'm Shelba," she says, pulling out a CD from her bag. "I was a drummer too, but I just started playing this a few years ago. They originated in Sweden and they're expensive."

We talk music, I explain the TAH, and she tells me she used to be a cardiac nurse. She gives me the CD – twenty songs of her original compositions. We trade info and Christie and I head back to the room. My frustration and anger from earlier has melted away. Music soothes the savage beast, I suppose. I agree to have the stupid PICC line moved yet again later that day, and the tech comes by to place the sheath right there in the room within a few hours. When Brehm wins an argument, he moves fast in case I decide to change my mind. Old German guys. . .

* * *

Everyone says that," Angie tells me. We're riding the elevator up to Christie's floor where I sometimes hang out at night if she's working. "Perry said it all the time." She doesn't look at me, just watches the lights on the control panel. "I got to be the one who told him that night."

Neither of us say anything until the doors open. I don't know if we're exhausted from talking about Perry, or if it's still too painful. Both, I guess.

"But it will happen," she says. "And I won't say, 'when you least expect it because all of you guys are way past the point of expecting it."

Angie is part of my tribe too. The N.P. office is directly across the hall from my door, so we often talk back and forth, and she checks on me from time to time – an actual gut check beyond the trite, "so how are you doing." They've got to be sick of hearing The Force Awakens over there by now, and the constant rotation of Firefly episodes emanating from the room.

"We are not going to die today, Bendis. And do you know why we're not going to die?" Captain Mal Reynolds asks the frightened staff sergeant, one of the three surviving platoon members boxed into the end of a canyon under heavy fire in the first episode of Firefly.

"Why?" Bendis asks, wide-eyed with terror.

"Because, we are so very, very pretty. We're just too pretty for God to let us die," Mal responds, before running wildly into open fire to bring down an enemy plane, then boldly losing the entire war.

Mal Reynolds, captain of the Serenity, narrator of all our hopes and fears.

Angie isn't afraid to talk about death, despair, shattered hopes. Attrition. She knows. We've spent a lot of nights sitting around talking about all of this.

"Biology isn't much beholden to hopes and dreams. But it's very fond of statistics," I said to her early on. She's a person of faith, to be sure, but also a realist. We hit it off immediately.

Of course, it's her voice at 3:30 am on May 24th, 2016, when my door slides open in the dark. Between the TAH and being isolated at the end of the unit in Room 1170, only the loud noises penetrate the solace at night. I was on the phone with Christie until two, and no one ever bothers me between 12 pm and 10 am. My door opening in the middle of the night can only mean one thing. And when I hear Angie's voice, I know, because an N.P. isn't going to come in for anything else.

She's very formal. She's been Angie, my across the hall buddy for months. Now she's 100% nurse practitioner. All business. I don't even sit up in the bed, I just wait to hear it, to soak in the words. She gives me the whole spiel.

"Mr. Johnson." Not Dave. Mr. Johnson. "We have a heart for you. It should arrive at the hospital around noon, you are scheduled for surgery at 2pm this afternoon. You should drink some water, because you are officially N.P.O. (no food or drink) as soon as I leave the room. Do you have any questions?"

On an hour of sleep? What else is there to ask? I know she can't tell me any of the things I've been wondering for four years. Seventeen in the back of my mind. What's his name? Did he have a family? How did it happen? How old? Married? Kids? Criminal? Social Worker? Pastor? Serial Killer?

"No," I say.

"Okay. I'll be back in with some paperwork once you've had time to get up and dressed. You should expect things to start moving really fast within the hour."

I nod. Once she's completely out the door, she turns into Angie again, spinning around and sticking her head back in.

"I told you it would happen! We were going to let you sleep but I figured you'd want to call Christie as soon as you could. Hurry. This is going to get crazy, fast."

I'm left alone in silence again. I need to call Christie. It's happened. Finally.

But this means I have to get another A-line in the wrist. I'm not sure how that's going to go, but they're going to need a few big guys to hold me down. Even connected to the big TAH machine, I can take out Dr. Pasad and Soleimani in the O.R. when someone goes to grab my wrist. I can do all the rest of this. I'm prepared. But I can't willingly give them my wrist again to stick that line in, knowing how bad it's going to hurt. It'd be like forcing yourself to stand still so someone can hit you in the face with a baseball bat. I don't have the willpower.

I call Christie. It's Tuesday morning, and she's planning to come up later today to help me bathe and to change the TAH dressing, our weekly ritual depending on her days off.

The clock says I just hung up with her a little over an hour ago, and she's already asleep, despite being a night owl from working third shift.

"Sorry to wake you up. I just wanted to tell you not to worry about coming up to change the dressing tomorrow. They've decided to just leave it off for good."

"For good? What are they going to do?" A few seconds of silence. "Are you getting a heart?"

"At 2 pm. Angie just came into tell me."

I don't remember what she said next, I just remember she had to get off the phone really quickly because she went and vomited.

The phone rings. "Sorry. I'm going to get a shower then call you back so you can tell the boys."

"You don't have to come right now."

"We want to be there. And there's a lot to do."

When the phone rings again, it's a groggy Rich. "Mom said you need to tell me something."

"I was just telling her she didn't have to change the TAH dressing today, because they're going to take the whole thing out."

"You got a heart?"

"Yep. 2 pm today. Are you busy?"

"Um...no. Wait. Let me check my calendar. No."

We laugh. Nervous laughter. So much of that lately.

"Dr. Soleimani is out looking at it now, but they don't have anyone else in line for it." More info from Angie between phone calls.

"I'm happy."

It takes Brennan longer to wake up.

"So, you get a heart? Today?"

"Yep."

"I thought so. You don't usually call us at this time."

"No more TAH," I say.

"No more TAH."

They're showered dressed, and in the room in about an hour. Fast. I've already seen Dr. Soleimani by that time, who apparently flew to wherever the organ was harvested and actually laid eyes on it.

"It is healthy. There are no antibody problems, no drug history. It's healthy, and a good fit, but no signs of HCM."

He sits on the bed and lays a hand on my arm. The stoic Indian man.

"I will not lie to you. What we are doing today puts every single one of my skills to the test. It is the hardest and most dangerous procedure that I do. I am good at it. But it is a very high risk. You could bleed to death. You could succumb to the anesthesia and not wake up. You could become paralyzed or have a stroke. There are many things that can go wrong. I don't have to tell you any of this, because you know. You were there."

Perry.

"I trust you," I tell him. And I do. I have. He got me here, safely.

"When I put in the TAH, I wrapped it in a material that should prevent a lot of the bleeding that Perry had. I have no worries about antibodies, but the wrap should cut down on the need for a lot of transfusions. It will take about five to six hours to remove the TAH correctly. We'll have to clean up, and it will be bloody, regardless. I have to do this right and be thorough. We've timed it so that once we're done with that, the new heart will be here, we'll have gone back over the blood work and history a third time, by a second team. So, lots of eyes and checks before we put it in. That will only take about two hours. You may be open on the table for a while if the timing doesn't line up exactly right, but you'll be on bypass, so it will be fine. I need to know that you are with me today. What is your feeling?"

Loaded question. "We've been on this path for a long time now. I'm not scared of the surgery, and I can't be anywhere else to have it done. I wouldn't be. We've all made good decisions up to this point. There's nothing else I can do. If it screws up now, it's on you, man. I'm not going to be around to worry about it."

He laughs out loud, probably the first time I've heard him do it.

"So, I have to deal with Christie."

"Yeah, I'm dodging that bullet. But good luck with that." I pat his arm.

"She will not be the only one angry, I think. This will be good motivation for me."

We're both in good humor. He knows that all anyone can think about is Perry. How can we not? But Perry wasn't his fault.

First, Christie and I make phone calls like crazy. Our parents. Then Marc Gecker and Michelle to come to the hospital to sign Do Not Resuscitate witness papers. No drastic life-saving measures, no veggie-keeper machines. I decided a long time ago that I can live with paralysis, but not without my mind. Christie knows all the details. We're interrupted dozens of times by the well wishes of every nurse, doctor, maintenance person, Intensivist, coordinator, and janitor. Despite HIPPA, word gets around fast; Christie and the boys are probably telling everyone they bump into on the way in. Hesitant excitement. We've all been here before, early in the morning on the HVI, hoping the day ends well. Our hope is tempered by the brutality and bitter terror of what happened that day. We decide to watch The Battle for Serenity Valley Firefly, Episode 1 to get our minds off it.

Mudgeman, and my first nurses, Natalie and Joanna pop-in, as does janitor Larry and Chuck, my separated at birth soul-brother. Tina comes in to connect me to the big machine, no pranks this time. She's happy to be done with me, says so, and gives me a big hug. I don't see Fran, the main person I want to see, but I know she's knee deep in paperwork, phone calls, and her typical whirlwind of activity when it's a transplant day. Right now, she's more concerned with vetting the new heart than my state of mind. If they miss something there, all the rest of this won't have mattered.

It all goes by so quickly. I'm saying my goodbyes to Christie and the boys (the standard Leia/Han Solo "I love you." "I know." thing). The hall is filled with everyone I've lived with for the last five months, like that final scene in Scrubs. Patients, nurses, physical therapists, the TAH team. There's Mudgeman and crazy Brian giving me the thumbs up and heavy metal signs, Brain with a proper Gene Simmons tongue hang. I smile and wave, the very picture of confidence.

Once we hit the hallway, I panic. Babbling to the prep team pushing the bed.

"Last time they said they had to place the A-line while I was awake because they needed numbers before and after sedation but this time they should be the same numbers because there's no margin for error everything is set on the TAH so it won't change so they should just be able to put me under then put the A-line in so that I'm knocked out because I don't think I can stay awake for it without them having to wrestle me down to put it in and I'm going to be fighting them, I know this about myself and if they miss, they'll have to try it again so it's probably better if they can figure out some way to put me down first, then put it in because I don't see why the numbers would change because the TAH won't be affected by the anesthesia, right? It shouldn't be because…"

They're not responding to any of this because they can't get a word in edgewise. My babbling continues all the way into the ER, where I can't even shut-up long enough to look around see who's there that I know. The prep team having fled from my frantic monologue the moment they moved me to the operating table, I direct my begging to Dr. Pasad. I know the drill here, he's supposed to calmly explain how this is going to go, be direct with me, then when the time for anesthesia comes, he's going to count down slowly from ten and everything will fade gently away around seven.

"...the TAH is controlling all that right?" I continue my babbling. "So, it won't matter, the numbers are going to be the same, so all around, it's better to just wait until I'm out to do the A-line, that way you're not having to fight me, because I know I can't do it again. I'm not worried about you guys or the surgery, but I can't do that line while I'm awake again, I just don't have it in me, I know my limits. I can even tell you the settings, check them on the pump if you want, they're-"

Blackness. Pasad didn't even count me down, he just hit me with everything he had, and I was out. I can imagine him now looking up at a bewildered Dr. Soleimani and asking, "What? He wouldn't SHUT UP."

I was in for about seven hours I'm told. It goes by like a quick catnap. Like closing your eyes during a TV commercial because you're so sleepy, but you just want to see the last two minutes of the show.

I'm in and out enough to recognize which room they're rolling me into. Same room I had on the side of the unit when I was admitted with the TAH back in January. What is this obsessive need to be oriented with my environment at moments like this? East wing, east side of the building, my bed facing southeast. I tuck that little tidbit away, note that I don't recognize any of the nurse's voices, don't see Christie, but they're telling me it went off without a hitch.

It's Dr. fricking Soleimani. Of course it went off without a hitch. But my right shoulder feels like I was kicked by a horse. Why doesn't anything else hurt? I fade again.

When I come back, Christie's there holding my hand, wearing a mask. I'm still intubated, but alert enough to understand my blood sugar is high and the heart is being paced but beating strong on its own. Tube will be out when I'm more awake. All good news, but I worry they dropped me from a table somewhere. My right shoulder feels like it's out of the socket. Such intense pain, but there's no way to really communicate this. Sleep takes me again.

I don't remember when the tube comes out or when I finally, really wake up. Christie says it was days. It feels like hours to me. I remember waving slightly to her and the boys through door. A few familiar nurse faces, but where are my normal people? I try to tell them about my shoulder several times, but no one gets it.

Two recurring dreams (hallucinations). My body must know it's hungry, though my stomach doesn't rumble. When I close my eyes, I'm presented with a digital touch screen that I can control with small nods of my head, or just by thinking about what I want it to do. A collection of chef resumes, listing credentials and details of their specialty dishes, most Italian, a few Indian. I spend a great deal of time in my head carefully weaning these down to three. One is Kim Dickens, who played a struggling Cajun chef named Jeanette Desautel on HBO's Treme, one of my all-time favorite shows. She's the one to beat. For what, I have no idea, but I feel like I'll be interviewing them for something later. The Indian chef has done something to make me rage-inducing angry. I have no idea what, but every time his face appears on the screen I'm filled with such hot-headed hostility, I can't go back to sleep (or am I already asleep?). It's all a hallucination, but each time I close my eyes, I see this same vision, thrown against my will back into this endless loop of chefs, entrees, until eventually, there he is again. It seems to go on for days.

The other hallucination kicks in when I do manage to open my eyes. I start to see familiar nurses walking by my open door. Their faces are the same, but they're all the average height of Willie's Wonka's Ompha-Loomphas and speak in high-pitched helium voices. I find this neither funny or disturbing, just curious.

And the shoulder pain, always the shoulder pain. I feel people changing bandages on my chest cold, hot, dripping, but no pain. My shoulder wakes me even from the drug-induced delirium, pervasive, persistent, and intense. I know they're giving me pain meds, but it's not touching my shoulder.

Finally, I'm awake enough to carry on conversations. Christie and the boys come in with masks. I just stare at them in wonder as the enormity of the whole thing hits me. Not just the transplant. All of it. The fruitless trips to St. Louis. Leaving the Ozarks packed into a van. The apartments, the moving, the contracts. Boston. Leaving Boston. The nightmare move to Lebanon, PA. The two and a half years of swans caths. Perry. The TAH. Perry. Living with the TAH. Perry died. Living in the hospital. A heart transplant. A single moment of clarity.

"What did we just do?" I whisper. Someone takes a picture and I'm out again.

Days blur by. I have a blockage and can't move my bowels. Katie inserts an NG tube up through my nose and down the back of my throat to suck anything and everything out of my stomach. It's incredibly painful and ironic that the task falls to Katie; Perry and I took to blaming her for literally any and everything that goes wrong on the unit as a running gag. Fridge broken? Katie's fault. Labs aren't back? Katie's fault. Docs clamped down on someone's fluid intake? Blame Katie.

It takes her two tries to get it in and the pressure makes my eyeball feel like it's popping out.

"We'll call this one my fault," she says, once the deed is done.

No water, no food, not even ice. This goes on for three or four days, and always, always, always, the intense pain in my shoulder. I think there's a broken bone.

The hunger and thirst eventually send me into on-and-off hallucinations again, mostly the chef database. In Stephen King's novel *Full Dark, No Stars*, the main character, "supposed that even in Hell, people got an occasional sip of water, if only so they could appreciate the full horror of unrequited thirst when it set in again."

I'm hot, I'm cold, Christie massages me as best she can, even soaking her hands in ice water at one point because I was so hot and couldn't cool off. She's exhausted and I'm hungry, getting angry if she leaves the room, the nurses say, because I suspect she's going to eat or get something to drink. I have no memory of any of this. I ask her to shave my beard, get angry when she does. Mudgeman comes to visit and I spend most of the time crying about something I don't remember. The steroids are having their way with me. I want to listen to music. It's the only thing that distracts from the thirst, hunger, and pain in my shoulder. Christie starts to realize that as emotional as some music makes me naturally, she has to skip over certain tracks because my violent sobbing risks bursting my chest incision. The worst is "June" by Spock's Beard, a band that captivated me several months ago and has been on no-stop rotation in Room 1170 to the point that even the nurses know the words to the songs.

> "June...came upon us much too soon, then was gone,
> Gone, like the mountains of the moon, at dawn.
> And the sun came up on a sleepy day
> and never went down at night,
> And the band going singing Waste Away,

*but it just didn't feel right,
And we knew, it couldn't be true...
it was free, but it wasn't for me..."*

(June – Spock's Beard)

I have no idea what some of the lyrics mean but I realize that June has come. In May, I wondered if I would ever see June. The TAH had been acting up and no one knew why. It had been nine months at that point, the period of time I'd given myself. I knew I could do nine months. Beyond that, for whatever arbitrary reason, I didn't know if I could keep going. I'd just made it to June, but it seemed too good to be true, like it was all happening to someone else. Every little part of this journey just seemed to end worse than it had begun, and I'm not yet ready to believe this would be any different, despite the assurances of everyone around me. This is chronic for transplant patients who feel they must, MUST put on a happy face for the excited people around them. They internalize their fears and worries about all that lies ahead. We're still at high risk for graft rejection, the new drugs are working havoc on our minds and bodies, and we're thinking about infection, the next biopsy, trying to walk again, our memories, pneumonia, and perhaps the scariest thing - what am I supposed to do now?

I've never been a healthy person. Not ever. I've had a congenital heart disease from the day I was born. I have no context or experience navigating life as a fully-functioning human being. And I'm terrified.

The song "June" seems to encapsulate all of this for me, and after the first post-transplant listen I break down in sobs that make my incision ache. Christie has to remove it from my playlist. Following it is a lot of U2, Goyte, Soilwork, Kip Winger, Bruce Hornsby, and Yes. My mood swings more violently than ever and nurses come into Appalachian bluegrass one hour and Swedish death metal the next (I would argue they're pretty much the same thing). I'm revisiting Mozart for the first time in twenty years and trying to devour a much-neglected Dean Martin discography at the same time. All over the place.

The steroids are causing my restless leg syndrome to act up worse than ever, so that even when I can fall asleep, it tickles and twists me awake. Christie stands at the end of the bed with my foot in hand, simulating walking movements to keep the twitches away so I can at least get five or ten minutes here or there. Ellen Gecker comes and takes me through a guided relaxation and hypnotherapy session which finally puts me to sleep a few hours before my first biopsy on the week anniversary of the transplant. Christie guards the doors as I sleep and won't even let the doctors in until I wake up.

I can honestly say I've not despaired of life the entire eighteen years this has all been going on. No matter how bad the situation, there was always hope. Hope of a new med, a new procedure, a new method of fighting. We always had a next step to take, and we had at least some control over how we'd handle it. There were choices, and good or bad, we knew the consequences of those could be dealt with.

On that Wednesday morning, once I awake from blessed sleep at the hands of Ellen, I have enough clarity to despair. I've had no food, water, or even ice for going on five days. The NG tube has rubbed my throat, the inside of my nose, and my upper lip raw, and there is no liquid relief from it. I hallucinate most nights about ice, Gatorade, and Mountain Dew, the king of all laboratory birthed concoctions. I start to understand how someone could become so desperate for water as to drink out of a toilet, or their own urinal. And I feel like a savage. I'm not carrying on conversations well, and when I do, I just complain about the hunger and pain in my shoulder. I am in despair, and for the first time I think, "I wish I'd just died on the table."

I've never wished for death, or even fantasized about it. But I know physical pain can push people to that place, and I have finally met my limit. There is no escape from the unrelenting hunger, thirst, pain, misery, and stasis. Nothing seems good, or like it ever will be again. I'm trapped, and my mind tells me that no matter what anyone says, I'm dying, and there's nothing anyone can do.

When Dr. Popjes comes to get me for the biopsy, I can only look forward to the sedation. I tell him I want a lot, because at least I can escape the pain for a little while. I wonder how much I can push them to give me. Maybe enough that I just don't wake up. Nah. Angel would never let that happen.

The biopsy is good, which helps a little, and the sedation was enough of a break in the monotony of pain that my wish for death flutters away that afternoon. Nothing helps my shoulder, or the gnawing hunger and thirst. I'm weak from it. Cassie is with me that day, patiently dealing with every little moan and groan, working like mad without breaks or probably lunch to do what she can. Before she leaves, I pat her cheek and tell her, "I'm glad it was you today." Her eyes well up and she doesn't know what to say. If I could have picked anyone on this, my worst day, it would have been Cassie.

***

Why it takes me an entire week to realize that my A-line (placed so graciously by Dr. Pasad after shutting me down with anesthesia) is in my right, not my left wrist, escapes me.

"Was this moved?" I ask. When? Why?

"It wasn't drawing back very well, so the doctor moved it while you were out a few days ago," Mem (Mary Ellen, my nurse) tells me. "Do I need to look at it?" she says lifting it up for a better view.

My stomach lurches and I scream so loud it startles even her permanently calm demeanor. "Does it hurt?"

"My shoulder," I groan. "It hurts my shoulder when

you lift it."

She puts a hand on my shoulder and lifts the wrist again. I writhe and bite down on a curse. Agonizing in the extreme. Now she's concerned. "Something may be wrong with this line. It's drawing fine, but I need to look at it."

She gets Victoria, our little South American comedian on the night shift to help her remove the bandage. I'm trying to stay still but each small removal of a layer of pressure is like someone stabbing me in the shoulder with a jagged icepick. When the final layer of gauze comes off, it peels with it two, one-inch long, inch deep chunks of flesh from the soft underside of my wrist. I gasp and nearly pass out. I hear the worry in Mem's voice. She leans into Victoria and says under her breath, "Uh-oh. Christie is not going to be happy about this."

I'M not happy about this, but the pain is so intense, all I can do is lay there and moan.

I've developed a horrific allergy to adhesive over the last year. Even band aids will cause me to blister and bleed after they've been on for a few hours. Christie, in her relentless pursuit to make all this work, discovered a skin prep solution called Cavilon. It's usually on hand, even in the hospital, unless you don't know where to look. We've used it underneath the PICC line and TAH bandage since the second month, because otherwise, anywhere tape or adhesive touches my skin, it leaves a blistered, bloody mess within two hours. My white blood cell count shoots up to fight the infection. Everyone freaks out because they worry my lines or the TAH cavity has become infected. No one knew what to do, but Christie solved it. It literally saved me from being stalled on the waiting list several times due to "unexplained infection risks."

When the A-line was changed from the left to the right wrist, this crucial piece of information was not passed along. Consistency of care failure. So, the bandage on my right wrist had been covering a thick layer of generic adhesive for nearly a week, and the problem was just buried in with the ups and downs of my ever-changing blood work numbers, rather than standing out like it would have a week earlier on the TAH. The skin assessment team finally proves their worth by showing up quickly with topical lidocaine for the pain, and a gel bandage to cool the spot and fill in the gaping holes in my flesh. This finally convinces the team to give me some pain meds, which at this point are being withheld in an effort to get my digestive system working. At last, my shoulder calms down, and I sleep for five consecutive hours, at night, without hallucinations of chef databases or Oompah-Loompahs. In the months that follow, my chest incision and TAH site in the abdomen start to heal, but the gaping abscesses on my wrist cause me more trouble and pain than those two combined.

The thought that occupies my every idle, lucid moment is obvious. What group of people, somewhere out there is coming home to a house with one less person? Who is going to work forced to look at that empty desk or chair? What wife is facing a closet or dresser that must be cleaned out? A car that he won't ever drive again? I've wondered about and grieved for this man and his family, his friends for so long, I feel like I know him. But I never will. He's a fictional construct I've used to process this idea that we will make a trade, one life for another. Not willingly on his part, or at least I hope. But either by purposeful will or simple goodwill in a snap decision, he decided to give what he could once the worst happened. Or his family decided to, after the fact, in that awful moment when the awkward question was asked. The thought that someone would even be able to consider such a thing with any presence of mind in such a moment fascinates and horrifies me. I don't think I would have the strength to do it myself. I hope I never have to find out.

I want to skip a year ahead in this story for a moment. Gift of Life, my local organ donor program allows organ recipients to write a letter to the family of their donor. Most never hear back. When I tell people this, they respond with a puzzled look. Surely the person who gave such an unthinkable gift would want to meet the recipient. Or would they?

There are at least a dozen reasons why they might not. There's understandable trepidation on both sides of this exchange. Everyone would love to think that the recipient of their loved one's liver, kidney, lungs, or heart is living life to its fullest, spreading joy, carrying the legacy of their loved one in a way that inspires and encourages everyone they encounter. Wouldn't it be easier to live with that assumption, than to meet the recipient only to discover that they're not a good person? That they're wasting the second chance they've been given? That they're hateful, mean-spirited, or even ungrateful? In one case that we know of, the recipient was Dick Cheney. Can you imagine?

As you'll see in the next few chapters, newly transplanted patients aren't really themselves for quite some time after the surgery. There are a lot of steroids playing tricks on the mind, and the psychological fallout from all that has happened takes a while to settle. There are no doubt stories circulating in donor support groups in which the survivors regret having made contact with the recipients.

On the recipient side, we'd like to imagine the same things. But for all we know, our donor might have been a terrible person. Possibly killed while driving drunk, or in a shoot-out with police. We have no idea. Isn't it possibly better to content myself with the fiction that they were a wonderful person who is remembered fondly? That if I ever were to meet his family, they'd receive me with open arms? What if they turn out to be drug addicts, alcoholics, dysfunctional, or resentful? The whole scenario is problematic.

It takes me an entire year to even know what to say to my donor family. One night, the following spring, out of nowhere, I suddenly sensed it was the right time. I sat down and wrote the letter in an evening, from notes I'd been editing in my head for years. The same is true of the lyrics to the song I recorded for my donor and his family - it came in a flash and I only changed one or two words by the time it was finished.

My letter to them better explains my thoughts and emotions about the whole thing than I can summarize here. I won't reprint the whole story I'm telling here, but the letter read in part:

I imagine every letter from a donor recipient to their donor family must contain so many cliché and trite phrases that fail at all to express or invoke the depths of emotion felt by either person. But I hope this is the only such letter I'll ever write, so please forgive me if I say things that I'm sure you've heard many times by now.

There is the obvious, and I'll state it bluntly; I would be dead were it not for this Thing that took place around May 24th of 2016. I'm thankful to you, to your loved one, for the incomprehensible sacrifice and gift that was given to me that day; I'm trying to repay it to everyone I encounter, but if I lived another hundred years, I'd not be able to repay it properly. A face that I cannot see, a voice I've never heard, compels me to repay that gift. I need that push, because I can be a real grump sometimes, and I fail to recognize how amazing life is, even at its worst. I carry inside me an inescapable reminder now.

To say I made it to transplant by the skin of my teeth is an understatement. There were so many bad things, the hard journey, the experience that I know no one will fully comprehend except the four of us who endured it. But here's the point: we did it all on a vague hope, just to have a chance. All of the sacrifice, upheaval, grief, anxiety, time apart, stress, and tears...it's my Story, my family's Story. For better or worse, it has shaped us and redirected our lives.

It's a difficult, and almost unbelievable Story, even for us who experienced it. But to my mind, it's not really the most important part of my transplant Story.

I'm still confused about a great many things in life, but I have absolute, crystal clear clarity about one single thing; that all of this that's happened to me, my Story, wouldn't be worth telling had not someone I'd never met, chosen to do a good thing, had his family not chosen to do a good thing at the worst moment of their entire lives. I've written nine paragraphs full of medical nightmare here, and it all would be pointless, for nothing, if it weren't for this stranger who I'll never meet.

I love stories. I've been an avid reader all my life, and I write a lot myself, so I tend to think about life in terms of stories. And that's just it, isn't it? This Story is really not about me or my family in the end – it's about that stranger. Without him at the end of the whole thing, there is no Story to tell. Not really. It would just be the sad tale of the married father of two, struck down in the middle of life by an unfortunate genetic mutation. It all would have been pointless, and I'd have spent the last years of my life dragging my family around the country in the vain hope that I could be saved. Do you see? It was really about him from the beginning, from the moment I was told I needed a new heart. That's when it became about him. Would that person out there, somewhere, whoever he was, do a good thing? With each day that passed, and that now passes, my whole Story – all of it; past, present, future – hinges on him, and on you. On what kind of person you are, what kind of person he was. I think about it every morning when I open my eyes. To me, that's the real Story. It's the story I am telling people when I talk about my transplant. He's the hero of the whole Story.

You are in the middle of your Story now, and no one will ever understand it but you – there are too many details, too many thoughts and memories that just can't be expressed with words. Loss is indefinable like that. Grasping at smoke, trying to describe it to others, until your heart and spirit become too exhausted and bereaved to talk anymore, and you finally realize that some things will be yours alone to keep, for better or worse, never to be shared with or understood by anyone else. My Story is full of such moments. I just figure the most valuable treasures should be hidden away, after all, right?

This time last year, sitting in the same hospital room for the fifth month, missing my family, wondering if these would be my last days, I fantasized about sitting on my front porch, drinking a glass of tea (drinking tea! I had a fluid intake restriction for 6 years!), feeling the breeze on my face as the sun sank behind the trees... and writing such a letter as this. I tried to imagine it, as a means of escape, because I was almost sure it would never really happen. I spend a lot of time sitting on my porch now, drinking as much tea as I want, usually until it's dark, staring at the trees and the sky and marveling that a near-dead man can feel so alive. I had my one-year biopsy last Wednesday and this heart is healthy, happy, and working hard to get the rest of my body in shape. I can't believe how active I can be now without pain and chronic fatigue. My boys are amazed too. We'll be taking a camping trip for the first time as a family in June, and we plan to do some hiking and canoeing. I've not been able to even consider such things since before they were born.

For so long it was hard to imagine or believe that there was any light, or goodness, or hope on the other side of all our panic and grief. Even believing it existed didn't chase away the darkness or heal the scars that we carried – I'm trying to accept that they are part of who I am now, that I will live with those bad experience for the rest of my life, that I will never "get over it." I'm not one who believes that time heals all pain. I think it becomes part of who we are. And if we're lucky, maybe it makes us more patient, more empathetic ... wiser. I hope so.

This letter could be so much longer, because there are so many things I want to ask you. I won't right now, because I fear I might be treading on yet-sacred ground. I've waited a year to write because it's taken me this long to even gain a small bit of perspective on what has happened between us, between me and this person to whom I, my family, my parents and brothers, and so many friends are now indebted.

It's also taken me this long because, what in the world do you say to the loved one(s) of the person who literally saved your life? I can't even bring myself to simply say "thank you." That's what you say to someone who holds the door for you or brings food to your table. It's not enough. Neither does it seem appropriate to gush on and on about how wonderful he must have been and how sorry I am that we had to meet in this way. It's too much.

If there's one thing I could hope for us both, for all of us, inexplicably thrown together because of a random mix of genetics, happenstance, timing, hope, and tragedy, is that we would have peace. I haven't known peace in mind or body for so long that I'm slow to recognize it even now. I know that your peace has been disrupted and wounded, permanently. But for me, any small bit of peace does more than "thank you," or platitudes about a loved one being in a better place, or all things having a greater purpose. I don't know if any of that is true or not, but I know that peace can sustain us until we figure it out.

I wish it for you, with tears of gratitude, and with utter grief for your loss. I wish it for me, trying to figure out where I fit in now, how to pick up the pieces of a life that's been on hold for so long that I almost forgot who I am. Peace is something I know can be found in the middle of any storm, no matter how much it rages around us, or how much we rage against it. I hope with all my being we can both find it somehow, in the midst of this Thing that has happened to us. I hope we have the chance to help each other find it.

Peace to you,

Dave, Christie, Rich, & Brennan

April 23, 2017

Chapter 18

The Other Side of the Sun

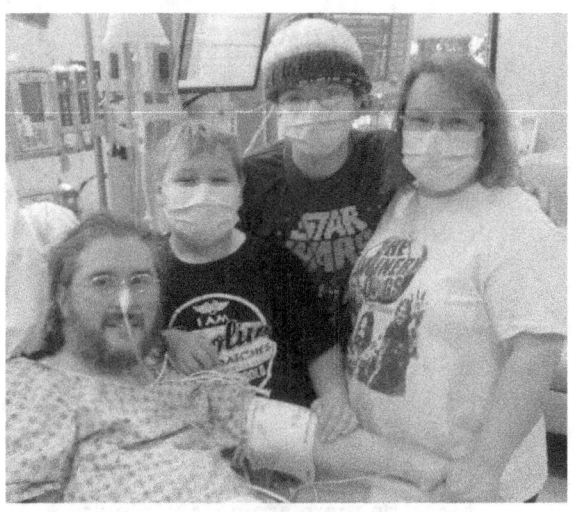

Waking up from the longest fever dream
Nobody knows the trouble I've seen
High again, then down in the gutter,
Euphoria, depression, the glory and the clutter

I'm on the other side of the sun (it's a brand-new day)
Back from the dead, what have we done?
(just might get away with this)
Standing where my shadow used to be,
the air is clean now we can breathe
Soak it in, we're free at last –
the other side of the sun, this side of the grass

Waking up to a truth I never knew,

Even if you survive regret can kill you
Half my life has passed me by,
Suspended, twisting, but now it's my time

Guess you just had to be there (no one can tell you)
One more go-round with the nightmare
(round and around and around)

Back in 2016 as the days drifted into nights and I finally started to gain some sense of time, the dawning realization that there might actually be a life beyond all of this is overwhelming. I'm still trapped in a bed with wires and tubes everywhere, but my mind is constantly racing, and I'm manic. I can almost taste freedom.

My digestive system wakes up and the NG tube comes out. This also means I can finally restart my restless limb medications, which in turn means I can sleep. I have a few lucid conversations with people over the phone - my parents, a cousin, friends, my in-laws, and Leslie. The nurses let a few people in the room to visit, and I actually get to see the boys for more than ten minutes at a time. Christie seems to be there around the clock.

I know things are turning around when I wake up a few mornings into the second week, needing to urinate like a normal human being, hungry, and looking for my laptop. I want to do something other than lay in the bed all day. There are letters to be written now - to doctors and others who have been pivotal in all of this. I'm also determined to leave my patient proposal for long-term care changes on the HVI in the hands of the unit manager before I'm discharged. A committee is forming to deal with the situations that have arisen from having mobile, cognitive device patients mixed in with the induced coma population of the HVI unit, and I've lobbied hard to be part of the patient side of that conversation, bringing both mine and Perry's voices to the table.

I have notes from dozens of conversations with him that have to be included. I owe him that.

Massive doses of steroids add urgency to any task, so I'm up and ready to go at 6:45 this morning, the worst possible time of day for any nursing staff other than 6:45 pm. Shift change. Reports are being given, last minute charting and instructions from doctors fly back and forth, and there's inevitably a crisis that draws a lot of the staff to a single room. I know this schedule. I've been living around it for several years now. But... steroids.

Before Jess, my nurse for the day, can even make it into the room, I've shuffled myself to the end of my bed, legs hanging off, looking out of my door to see if I can get someone's attention. I avoid the call light, because rationally, I have no emergency. But... steroids, particularly high-doses of Prednisone, create a persistent "now or never" itch on the brain. I've been in and out of the bed a few times on my own strength, but I'm a fall risk. The impulse to act overcomes my good sense, and I manage to half-lean, half-stumble the two feet from the end of the bed to the chair, where my laptop awaits. Jess is not amused when she comes in the door. I don't know her well, but it sets the tone for the next few days. She barely leaves me alone and insists on helping me do things I'm already able to do by myself. We end up driving each other crazy.

I've got one letter finished when she brings food.

"Not much, because your system is still slow." She lifts the plate cover and for all the complaining about the terrible hospital food over the last half-year, this looks like a gourmet feast. Limp toast, mushy cubed potatoes, and cherry Jell-O. I don't even like Jell-O, and I'm absolutely not a fan of cherry-flavored anything, but the top is off and I'm shoveling it down without a thought.

"This isn't bad," I tell Jess as she busies herself with setting up my morning meds. "I've never really liked cherry much. It's okay I guess. It's always one of those flavors I tolerate. Three flavors of popsicles in a box, ya know? Orange, lime, and cherry - I'll always pick cherry last."

Prednisone makes you babble about the most irrelevant and mundane things as if they were the news of the year.

"Mmm-hmm," she says distractedly, her back turned. I think she's used to steroid addled post-surgery ramblings and I've already bombarded her in the short half-hour we've been together.

"I don't know why I do that," I say, scraping every little bit out of the plastic container. "It's not like it's a bad flavor. I guess I just decided when I was a kid that I didn't like it as much as the others, so I never even think to try cherry flavored things anymore." I fiddle with the toast a little, but a tide of emotion rises up and I burst into tears. "It's not fair, I know. I should just try cherry more often it, give it a chance. There's probably a lot of really good cherry flavored food out there that I've just ignored…"

I'm literally sobbing in guilt over my neglect of the flavor cherry. And a little bit over my well-known disdain for Jello in general ('non-food' I call it). Jess lays her hand on my shoulder. "So . . . do you want me to take it away, or . . . do you want some more . . . ?"

"Maybe it's because I've always liked strawberry more and if there are two red colors of something, I'll just pass over the cherry. I need to stop. Think," I cry. Jess hands me the tissues and I try to pull myself together.

"Why don't you just eat the toast. You haven't had any toast in a while," she says, an obvious effort to distract me from my existential crisis over the cherry Jell-O.

"I'm sorry," I say, my brain catching up with itself. "It's the steroids, huh?"

"It's the steroids," she says.

It's funny to me by the next meal, but I have no idea how telling this small moment of introspective nonsense is. In the year to come, I struggle by the minute to pull myself back from this type of piercing examination of every action I take in life, my motives behind it, and all possible consequences, realistic or fantastical. It becomes a paralyzing anchor that plagues me constantly.

Before I even leave the hospital, I've planned several music projects, written a ton of outlines for new books, and am surfing Craigslist almost hourly looking for drum sets, mixing consoles, guitars, and a dozen other things I can't afford. Terri Mudge warns Christie to keep my debit card away from me. She left for work one day after Mudge's transplant and came home to a new boat in the driveway. Steroids cause compulsion in even the most self-disciplined people. Overspending, over-committing, over-emoting. Everything is 100% or it's nothing at all.

The docs want me to go home, even though the drugs have caused excruciating neuropathy in my feet to the point that I can't walk without assistance. They're anxious to get me out of here, away from the germs and constant traffic of my hospital room. These last days seem to drag on forever, me frustrated with the painful swelling in my feet, unable to put weight on them much at all.

I don't drink coffee much, but the craving is insatiable right now. I can't have it the way I want it because of my blood sugar, but that doesn't keep me from begging the nurses for it constantly. I sit in my chair and yell, "COFFEE!" out the open door at any passing nurse until they just quietly close it. I badger Sonja, one of my NP's so much for it that she disappears for a bit, then hurriedly sneaks a small frap – no sugar, no cream, onto my table and rushes out. "I wasn't here," she whispers over her shoulder as she ducks out. Sonja's another member of my Village. Has been for a few years now.

Conversations from Room 1170

This room is way louder than 1170, across from the main nurse station, near the main doors to the unit. I don't sleep well. There's a guy down the hall threatening violence if the nurse doesn't give him back his pants. It's 2:30 in the morning and after lying awake listening to this for several hours, I finally page Adam. "He can have my pants," I tell him, motioning to my sweats hanging on the end of the bed. "Just give the guy some pants. Any pants."

"He's a WWII vet and he's delirious. He's still wearing the pants he came in with. He wouldn't let us take them without trying to hurt everyone," Adam says. "I've offered to give him another pair to put on over them, but they're 'not his pants.'"

"Oh," I say with a yawn. I'm wide-awake now, realizing how much of this nighttime noise I must have missed from being in 1170 at the end of the hall. "Can I get some coffee then?" I venture.

"No, Dave," Adam sighs wearily. "We've already done this today. Twice. No coffee. No caffeine. Go to sleep."

"Can I at least get my pants back, then?"

He gives me the finger and leaves the door cracked.

"COFFEE!" I yell after him.

Fifteen minutes pass and I'm still awake. And still craving coffee. I call the hospital operator and ask for an outside line to call back into the HVI.

"Sir, you can just dial the extension from your room," she tells me.

"Oh, I know. But I'd rather use an outside line." She doesn't ask questions.

I can hear the phone ringing at the desk outside my room as I wait for someone to pick up.

"HVIC, this is Adam."

"Yes, this is Dr.... Coffee," I say doing my best to disguise my voice. "I need someone to get a large Vanilla Mocha to room 1178, stat. There were orders given this afternoon, but it looks like they were missed at shift."

Adam is silent for a moment. When he speaks I can hear him in stereo through the phone and the door.

"Dr. Coffee," he says flatly.

"Yes, um, Dr. Coffee. From nutrition. I spoke with…what was her name, Jess, the day nurse this afternoon."

Another silence, then: "……Dave?"

"Um, no. No, this is Dr. Coffee. From nutrition." I know he's puzzling over how, and why, I'm calling from an outside line. The phone goes dead in one ear as I hear the desk phone slam down outside in the other.

"DAMMIT, DAVE, GO TO SLEEP!"

On this much Prednisone? I have to keep myself entertained somehow. The guy keeps yelling about his pants, which turns the whole unit into a circus for the rest of the night. Everyone's punchy, laughing, racing desk chairs around the inside of the nurse's station, goofing around. It's the first time I realize that as badly as I want to go home, I'm going to miss these guys and this place in some weird way.

Perry's family comes to visit the day before I leave. We cry a lot, or at least I do, unable to reconcile my relief at surviving the surgery with the guilt I feel that he didn't. His mother gives me the cane that used to stand in the corner of Room 1170 when he lived there. His favorite uncle made it for him, and I certainly needed something to prop me up. It felt right to take this small possession of his with me when I left, like he was helping me finally make my way out of the door after all this time.

Conversations from Room 1170

And finally, there's Fran, my coordinator, leaning in the doorway, her arms crossed in that "I told you so," manner she has.

"Well, kiddo, what did I say?"

"You were right. I know."

She nods, satisfied that I've admitted she was right. I did get through it. She didn't let me down. She won't tolerate any gushing or weepy thank-you's. Meds are straightened out, we get through my discharge medications, and Christie packs up what little is left in the room while I go for my two-week biopsy. All my stuff from Room 1170 is already back home, and I know she's been cleaning the house like mad with the help of friends to prepare for my triumphant, or at least exhausted, return...

In the ambulance bay where Christie pulls in to pick me up, Blake, ever present ball cap on his head, TAH thumping away, comes bouncing up with his wife.

"Oh! Glad I caught you! They said you were leaving today, so I figured you'd be back here."

I've never seen Blake not happy. He always seems like he's on the way to see his favorite ball team or claim a sweepstakes prize. I don't remember much of the exchange in the fog of waning sedation and exhaustion. I just remember how happy he was that I was safely on the other side. Rich, along with Perry's cane, help me into the car, and we're off. We stop on the way home to get Big Gulp slushies in his honor.

I mostly stare at the sky all the way home. The oft-jailed characters on my favorite TV show, The Wire, always tell one another, "There's only two days. The day you go in, the day you come out."

It's been one hundred and thirty-five days since the EMT's rolled me into the ER. Nearly eighteen years to the month that my HCM started to progress back in 1998. I feel older than any passage of time. So tired. But the four of us, together still, ride

Dave Johnson

along the two-lane road to our little space in the world. I just want to get there and close the door for a while.

Chapter 19

9-2-9

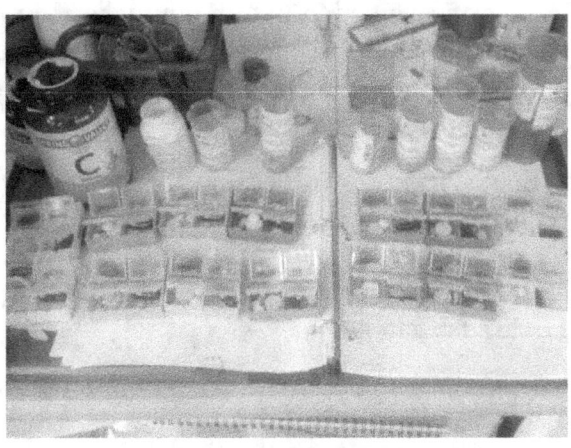

One more alarm bell, another scream in the night
One more exclusion, another do it or die
Tilting at clock towers, I'm the Don Quixote of time
Like an addiction, like nothing in me is mine
Gotta get around the bend, I'll choke it down until then

Nine to nine, poison wine, on my dime
Rain or shine, compliance line, nine to nine

Another shutout, another number to dread
The syndrome Stockholm, this powder's burning my head
This mad concoction, this venom keeps me alive
My brain on auction, losing my mind just to survive
Tweaking like a rock star on leave, no other tricks up my sleeve

My first few days at home are filled with just what I'd told everyone they would be.

"A shower, crab legs, then...drums."

I will never take the power of pressurized water for granted again. Between the TAH and the surgery, I've gone a few days short of ten months without much else than a sink bath. When the water hits my skin, it stings like needles, and I have to ease my way into the stream slowly. My muscles twitch and the heat is glorious. My back spasmed for half-an-hour when I first sat down on our couch, but the shower seems to work out a lot of the tension from the uncomfortable bed and chair I'd been trading between these last five months.

I'm finally in my own bed, no plastic covered mattress beneath the sheets, no light flooding in at the top of the doorway, no distant sounds of bells and voices. Just the sounds of cars passing, the occasional pop and settle of the old wood floor or furnace, or a dog stretching out.

I don't sleep long because hunger gnaws constantly. The pangs are persistent and cramp inducing; food doesn't stop them because they aren't really from hunger - they're caused by the Prednisone. Christie finally resorts to packing a small cooler and keeping it at my bedside. I can't get up and down the stairs, or to the bathroom really, without help. I know she's worn out beyond my understanding, so if I'm hungry - or my ever-turning brain awakes me before she's up, I try to lie there, eat quietly and let her catch up.

Regardless, we both have to be up and functioning by nine o'clock, and so it will be for the rest of my life. Anti-rejection meds run on a twelve-hour cycle and have to be reintroduced to the system at that interval to keep white blood cells from attacking the new organ. I can fudge a little on biopsy days, but no matter whatever else is going on in life, my day is bookmarked by two nines. AM and PM.

And it's complicated. At the start there are over seventeen separate medications that have to be taken at five different times each day, not counting some that have to be taken immediately before or after meals. This will change over time, but I'm experiencing frequent bouts of short-term memory loss, so everything is written down, programmed into my phone app with alarms, checked off, and double checked to make sure nothing is missed. I take vital signs, check my blood sugar every morning and night, and track everything to be reviewed by Fran and the docs at my weekly appointment. It's too much for my steroid-addled brain to keep up with, but Christie works to help me understand it all and I want fervently to be independent enough that she doesn't have to. I'm ready to do things for myself again.

Next: crabs. We meet Mudgeman and his wife, Terri, a few nights after I get home at a seafood place near their house. Crab legs, my favorite food, are scarce in land-locked Pennsylvania, but Jane and Dave's have all you can eat. They probably didn't account for me in that deal.

"Sanitize," Mudge says, about ten different times throughout the meal. Every time I touch a pepper shaker, or the back of a chair. Drink from a straw. Sanitize the silverware. Watch the waitress - make sure everything is as clean as it can be within your power. It's a good tutorial, and we all share a shorthand that makes it easy to be around each other.

Terri watches in amazement as I decimate the blue-crab population of the Eastern seaboard. After a few pounds of crabs and legs, I'm an hour in and not slowing down. She looks over at the scrap pile and asks, "Are you even starting to get full?"

"A little," I say between mouthfuls. I've dreamed of this moment for months. We take a picture of the destruction and send it to Fran, who will yell at me later about the salt. I just think it's incredible to be able to eat salt and not go home worried I may drown in my own fluid tonight. What strange new world is this?

Later that week, I find a drum set on Craigslist - the exact same make and model I sold back in 1998 when I first got sick. It was my dream kit and the transaction had been painful. I get it for a steal, and spend the evenings getting my chops back once Christie leaves for work. I catch up on all the King's X and Jellyfish albums I never got to learn. A spin through The Beatles "Help!" and "Rubber Soul," leaves me in awe (once again) of Ringo Star. It's going to take some serious study to even get close to imitating his feel and swagger. Underrated doesn't even begin to cover it. The man is a genius.

It's six weeks before I'm allowed to drive, so I'm home most of the time, monitoring what's left of the boy's school year, trying to get back into the habit of cooking and cleaning. Picking up where I left off for the most part. As a matter of principle, my first project is to finish painting the bloody trim in the sun room. The paint can is still there from the day I was rushed to the hospital back in January. Finishing the job is a personal triumph. Today, my desk sits directly in front of the spot where I thought I was going to die that day.

But the drugs slant and warp everything. The Prednisone especially has a way of digging deep into my worst doubts and fears about myself. Overthinking every decision, torturing myself over every misspent hour. I'm hyper-sensitive to anything or anyone who wastes my time, and critical of myself when I don't spend my free moments doing something productive. It's a common experience for transplant patients, and it makes sense; someone died and I'm alive as a result. What would their families give to have them back? It's a disservice to my donor to waste my days watching junk television and playing video games. As a result, I stay as busy as possible, trying to find ways to bring as much meaning into my daily routine as I can.

Christie, Brian, and Mudge warn me to pace myself - balance, patience, take time to rest or you'll burn out. Relevant points, but the medications exacerbate and amplify this drive to be busy, to DO something, now that I'm free from the shackles of HCM and the TAH. Perry is ever on my mind. He would certainly be pursuing his post-transplant aspirations with the same determination he had to survive. And that thought looms over me daily, not as a healthy check when I get lazy, but like a whip at my back, unrelenting. I find it hard to sleep much because I'm eager to start a new day. But until I can drive, there's only so much I can do at home, so I'm frustrated with my confinement. I begin to feel like I'm right back where I was with the TAH - trapped, immobile, stagnant. Six weeks seems like a lifetime, but my impatience and malcontent has more to do with Prednisone and Prograf in my system than with reality.

***

Brian is faithful to take me to lunch a few days a week and we talk about meds a lot. Where does my personality end and the drugs begin? Is this just the new me, post-transplant, and I have to find a way to reel in the excessive thoughts and obsessive need to be active every waking hour? Neither of us really know. The only thing that's clear is that whatever is happening, it's our life now. We're on a twelve-hour schedule that we can't break. Anti-rejection meds at 9am. Anti-rejection meds at 9pm. Nine to nine. When he, Mudgeman, and I are together at those times of day, our phone alarms startle everyone around us by ringing at the same time.

929 (Nine-to-nine) is the first song I write on this side of transplant. Those first few weeks, I consider the possibility that I have no songs left, that maybe the whole idea of writing songs is childish and it's time to move on to grown up things (like what? Doing taxes and complaining about the DOW? Who is Dow, anyway? What do grown-ups do?) The drugs tell you that everything you do is stupid, a waste of time, that you're a laughing stock for doing it.

But 9-2-9 comes busting out in a single sitting, finished without much need for re-writing or tweaking. It's loud, aggressive, and angry. More songs start to pour out, and I'm able to articulate so many of the complicated emotions I'm having. This is the way I always process change and struggle. Added to the songs I've written since all of this started in 2010, I have enough to fill two entire albums. The thought of a recording project is daunting; I just finished post-production on Instead of Wither in March while in the hospital, and I've got a dozen things left to do to promote my latest novel, Lorenzo the Magnificent. I don't have the equipment to record an album by myself, and I don't know any other musicians around here. I don't even know if I have the chops, instrumentally or vocally to pull something like that off. But I have the songs, and I need to tell this story. Maybe by telling it, I work through this "PTSD" I've been told to expect.

PTSD is a mystery to me - something that happens to soldiers or victims of violent crime. But I remember the panic attack I'd had at my brother's house several years ago. The same fight or flight sensation starts visiting me when I'm in a crowd or overwhelmed with stimuli. One afternoon Christie and I sit at the table in our sunroom, traffic flying by outside, the sun shining through the windows, the boys talking in the next room. We're trying to sort out medications and I realize I'm rocking back and forth, muttering, "too much, too much." Suddenly I'm frantic. Another panic attack? Christie gets me to a recliner and brings my noise cancelling headphones. I eventually fall asleep listening to The Beatles *Abby Road*.

The subsequent crashes are detoxification nightmares. Migraines, nausea, exhaustion without the ability to sleep, the inevitable worsening of the sinus infection I've been nursing since the week I left the hospital. The Methyl-Prednisone shreds my immune system, so there's no chance of fighting off even the least threatening of infections or common cold. The resulting biopsies blur together.

Through all of this, the medications are tweaked and adjusted. One particularly memorable two-week period has my skin crawling night and day, and everything hurts. I mean everything. Light, noise, the bottoms of my feet touching the floor. Pulling my pants on every morning feels like dragging a cheese grater over my legs. I sit on the couch staring into nothing and notice that when I inhale, the slight movement of my t-shirt against my skin hurts. I'm being weaned from the Prednisone and the accounts I've heard are not wrong. It's the worst thing I've ever endured, physically or psychologically.

One afternoon during all of this, Rich is putting away dishes. In my detox haze, I spin around and smash my left shin into the lowered dishwasher door. I know it's bad immediately because I can feel the blood running down my leg. Apparently, the Prednisone makes skin thin, and with all the fluid I've retained during the surgery, it was ready to burst. I'm left with a business card-sized patch of raw flesh, the top layer of skin torn away. It wasn't the worst scrape in the world, but when Christie tries to clean it, I scream at the top of my lungs, writhing in pain, while Rich physically holds down my leg. The tape burns on my wrist have to be irrigated as well so Christie just gets it over with. The pain is blinding, and I fall into a hard sleep for several hours after. We learn a few days later that the Prograf level in my blood is around twenty-seven - over twice what it should be, meaning I'm toxic and over immunosuppressed. The heightened reaction to pain, noise, and light suddenly make sense. It takes a few weeks to get my levels back down, and it feels like withdrawal again.

***

I'm working through some Bruce Hornsby tunes on the drums, trying to get my left hand in shape when I get a call from Rebecca, one of the new transplant coordinators.

"Hate to tell you this, but your biopsy from Tuesday showed rejection. 2R."

The very word "rejection" causes people to freak out. But this is more television show conditioning. Transplant patients know to expect this. Our coordinators tell us that everyone has rejection at least once. 1R (level one rejection) is a good result from a biopsy - it means the heart is healthy, yet there is still some agitation, indicating that the immune-system isn't completely suppressed to the point of being neutropenic, where you can and will catch anything floating in the air with no defense whatsoever, because the white blood cells are essentially sleeping on the job. A 2R result isn't terrible but has to be treated. Anything higher than that causes a great deal of concern, but the type and severity of rejection can range wildly within those numbers. My 2R appears to be mild, but it lands me in the hospital for three days on IV Prednisone.

Such is my history with Hershey Med Center and the HVI that I don't even have to be processed through the normal registration protocols when this happens anymore. I drop the van off, grab my "bug-out pack" (replete with a few changes of clothes, toiletries, ear plugs, noise cancelling headphones, laptop, current book I'm reading, and some snacks - my emergency hospital bag), and walk directly to a pre-assigned room on the HVI. Admission and registration comes to me, and I'm with familiar nurses who aren't happy, but not surprised to see me there. I go through the routine of unpacking and setting the room up. Once the IV is in, I make the rounds to see everyone.

Christie comes to see me before starting her shift and drops off a cooler with food for a few days (always faithfully helping me avoid the hospital food). Nurses and docs drop by to say hello over the three days, and Brian and Mudge show up together the second night and stay past visiting hours. We laugh, joke, and pester the nurses until lights out.

The Prednisone hits hard. At home I struggle with 10 mg oral daily. Here, it's 1000mg per day, IV. My brain doesn't slow down for about five days after, so even when the treatment is over, and I go home, I'm miserably tired but can't sleep. It lends an incredible amount of energy the first week or so, and I can be extremely productive, working at breakneck speed on music, my book, projects around the house, and seem to cram every second full of something on my to-do list.

Then the crash comes. Sleepy all the time, to the point that it's unsafe to drive. Nausea, migraines, skin crawling, blurred vision, and emotions out of control. Crying, hysterical laughter, intense anger over the most minor of things. It hurts to sit, it hurts to lay down. I wander around in a restless haze most of the time, settling for a few moments to work on some random task only to be distracted by some other thing that needs doing.

Christie and I were part of a study last year in which we discussed and answered questions about end of life decisions in various scenarios. In the end I had decided I would be okay living in a wheelchair, and possibly okay with impaired speech or vision. The two things I could not live with: deafness and loss of cognitive function. To not be able to hear music is to me a sentence worse than death. It would be like having my soul ripped out. To not be able to recognize my family or communicate with them, dependent on them for every life-sustaining action, and them subsequently trapped caring for me…that would be a living hell, made even more hellish by the fact that I wouldn't know I was living in it. The burden and effect on the boy's lives wouldn't be worth it just to keep a shell of me around.

Detoxing from Prednisone feels one step away from losing the ability to think rationally or make informed decisions. Things fly in and out of my brain so fast I can't keep track of them all, but I'm too tired and sick to even care, which is also frustrating because the creative side of me doesn't want to lose any melody, turn of phrase, or idea that pops into my mind.

Eventually, it's out of my system, but the nine-to-nine life continues. And it always will, until someone finds a better way to convince my white blood cells that the organ keeping me and them alive isn't a foreign invader intending harm.

About four months post, I end up in rejection for a third time. Prednisone won't do the trick. I'm admitted for three days to receive a drug called ATGAM. It's derived from horse serum, and because many people have nasty reactions to it, I have to take a pre-dose mix of Benadryl, Prednisone, and Tylenol. Benadryl has a history of keeping me awake for days, and the Prednisone...well, I've already been through that. Then the ATGAM in three doses over three days. I know I had visitors. Brian, Mudge, Marc and Ellen Gecker. But I don't remember much of anything. I stare at the wall a lot and take the opportunity to listen to Pink Floyd. I've always been told they make more sense if you're altered. At the time I enjoyed it, but I've tried listening to them since and I still don't get it. The rejection is gone on the next biopsy, the nine-to-nine meds are adjusted, and I make it through the holidays without incident.

"This is will be the easiest part, in the end," Perry told me back then. "Just waiting. The harder part is going to be after."

I don't know how he knew, but he did.

Chapter 20

Six of One

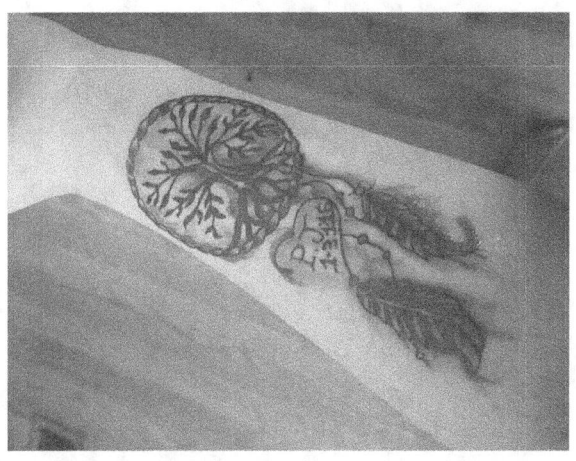

*She went home and died today
Probably someone else's mistake
Might have happened anyway
But who's to say - who's to say?*

*He was there when I went home
Still not himself, still pushing me along
His own fault, his self-abuse
No other excuse, no other excuse*

***Six of one, half a dozen of another
When we're gone, does the reason even matter?***

Conversations from Room 1170

Six of one, half a dozen of another,
Fate or sin, either way, I'm lost again

Back and forth, up and down
King of the hill with a tilted crown
Rebounds and fury, he sent us away
Saw the future, knew it was better that way

I can't seem to find a way forward,
but now there's no turning back
Trapped in the same vicious circle,
stumbling and falling off the track
Standing alone on this slippery surface,
watch as the rain crashes down
Clutching at hope, but it mocks me today,
pointing and laughing out loud
He told me to stare the thing right in the face,
but I can't even open my eyes
What does it matter when we've come so far,
just to fall at the very last mile....

Blake died last week.

He had a fidgety way about him, a slight bounce to his posture, even when standing in one place. I always imagined it was his unfettered energy that powered the TAH, rather than the Freedom Driver he carried in the backpack, long before I did.

He stuck his head in my room the day before I had my own TAH implanted. Five years older than me, his ever-present Redskins ball cap bobbing almost imperceptibly above his short frame. Where Perry was calm and quiet, Blake talked to everyone, his optimism and energy infectious.

"You'll get used to it," he said, grabbing his cannulas, as I would later grab my own out of habit. I believe it's an unconscious gesture that reassures us the thing stitched into our abdomen, attached to the device in our chests, is still there, still working. The way he jerked at his and flapped them around made my stomach turn at the time. But he was right. You get used to it.

He lived with the TAH twice as long as I did. The waiting list evaded him for a long time because he had liver issues that made him a bad candidate. Once he was listed, he got a heart. But his body rebelled against one of the anti-rejection medications, and he never made it home to his wife and teen-aged twins. He's the fifth fellow TAH patient and the fourth friend with a TAH that I've lost this year. I'm glad the boys didn't know him- I don't know how much more of this stuff they can take.

Yeah, the fifth. Did I mention that Jamie died a few weeks after she got home from her transplant? They transferred her to a hospital in Philly for the surgery and she did great. Went home to her two girls and her mom. She was separated from her husband, but he was ever present around the HVI, helping with the girls and talking to everyone. Where I had Christie, and most of the other transplant people I know are married with a spouse to do the aftercare and babysitting, she didn't really have anyone to do dressing changes and such, so a home health nurse came to her house to do wound assessment and dressing care. It was only a small cough, but that nurse went to work that morning anyway, to Jamie's house. Jamie died the next week from pneumonia, too atrophied and immunosuppressed to fight it off. I never heard what happened to the nurse.

And just like that - poof.

Perry worried obsessively about her not eating, but that kind of disorder is tough to beat. I had groceries delivered all the time to the HVI so I could cook in my room. I always tried to get a few of those disgusting microwave pizzas because they were one of the few things she would actually eat. And God forbid there be any kind of meat on the things. When the freezer started to fill up with them, I knew she wasn't eating them anymore. I'd catch Krista coming out of her room some nights with the food tray and she'd just give me a dark look and carry it off to the trash. Jamie became sullen if either Perry or I preached too much about her needing her strength for after the surgery. I think when he died, she pretty much gave up. If he couldn't make it, what chance did the rest of us have? She asked me that, the day after they changed her over the to the Freedom Driver, and the fill numbers wouldn't stop jumping around. I had no answer for her.

Brian told me about Blake as we left the hospital after the first meeting of a committee that's exploring ways to help long-term patients endure the wait. My reaction was pretty visceral - I doubled over on the sidewalk and just stood there for a few minutes, like someone had kicked me in the stomach. Brian leaned down and put an arm on my shoulder until I caught my breath again.

I should have spent more time with him, says the demon, regret, sitting on my shoulder. His wife managed the Dairy Queen in Palmyra and with him on the TAH, he had to be near someone trained on the equipment, so he spent his days sitting in a booth there, reading and surfing the web. I drove by there a lot on my way back and forth to the hospital. I could have dropped in to say hello, spent some more time with him. But being around a TAH patient was the last thing I wanted to do now that I was free. Selfish. But he would have known that and probably shoo-ed me away if I'd come in there anyway.

"You know being on this committee means we're going to get close to more people that we'll lose in the end," Brian said.

I just nodded and we headed to our cars.

"Perry and I had a deal," I said. "I'm going to keep it, as far as it depends on me."

We didn't say much more. I took the long way home that day.

***

Being chronically sick with heart disease thrusts you into relationships with people who also play knock-and-run at Death's door. But He's ancient and wise to that game. He catches people who you foolishly imagined were too quick and clever for him. I recite their names often. Joe. Dot. Perry. Jamie. James.

Blake.

Morbid as it is, Death has become an invisible friend, and He's no longer an enemy to me. It's nothing personal, He's just doing his job. But His constant brooding in the corner is intimidating nonetheless.

Everyone says I have survivor's guilt. Maybe? I don't know what that looks like, so I won't argue. All I know is I don't have the tools to withstand and absorb even more loss than I already have. My donor, to Perry's sisters and mother (especially), Jamie's little girls. Jame's wife and girls, Blake's wife and kids.

I think often of Perry's distinction between fear and courage. "They look exactly the same," he'd say. "But is it really courage when the alternative is dying? That sounds more like fear to me."

I'm not a courageous person, though people often insist that I am. My fears are many. I suspect that exposing myself to more death and loss will take a measure of courage that I've not yet discovered. I hope it's inside me somewhere, or that I can draw it from my family and friends. To live in a state of fear is a terrible thing, but it must somehow go hand in hand with hope and courage. I don't think it's a well you draw from that can be replenished. I think you just have to live as a broken person to empathize with broken people. And brokenness is harder than overcoming fear or being courageous.

Conversations from Room 1170

In the days that follow I get bits and pieces of information about Blake's liver not handling the Prograf, and other complications that finally got him. But much like the details of Perry's cancer, I don't really care. Maybe their families do. I guess I would if it were Christie or one of the boys. Dissecting the cause at that point does nothing to blunt the futility of it all.

This is why I hate post-game analysis worse than I hate actual football games. Replaying each and every success and failure with endless commentary on what the person chould or should not have done, where they went wrong, ad nauseum. At least in those circumstances the coaches can go back and assess problems, make corrections, and instruct the players to concuss each other differently the next time. What's to be gained from knowing the details of Blake's liver failure or Perry's cancer, or Jamie's pneumonia for that matter? What exactly is the lesson there? That someone can suffer for years, all through their childhood even, losing any chance of having anything that resembles a halfway normal life, do all the right things, pay for their sins, weep, pray, hope, wait, get cut on, cut up, poked, stabbed, prodded, bruised, and burned out only to die anyway? There is no lesson in that. Only despair.

I'm so desperately tired of people telling me everything happens for a reason. They can never exactly say what that reason might be. Only God knows? I've tried for years and can't square with the idea of a loving God who allows children to suffer, while yet having the power to stop it. It seems like negligent parenting at best, sadistic at worst. I used to think the same thing - "there's a purpose for everything." And I've watched individuals and families crumble and fall to ruin, addiction, suicide, and endless heartache waiting to see what that purpose is. My only answer is suffering. The purpose seems to be suffering. I've come to a point where I'd rather it be at the hands of cruel fate, or random chaos, than at the hands of a loving God. Because I don't know what to do with a God like that. I can't fathom allowing my children to suffer and standing back, doing nothing. What kind of parent would I be? If I'm powerless to intervene, whether by rules of my own or someone else's making…I don't know. That doesn't sound all-powerful to me. I know that many wise people have said "God is Love," but does that also mean that God is cruelty? After all, He does claim to the be the God of good and evil, darkness and light. For me, reconciling cruelty, suffering, or neglect, with love makes no sense, so I just steer clear as much as possible. The threat of eternal hell as a consequence for my lack of ability to figure that out or to just ignore the injustice of it seems only to prove the cruelty. It seems to me schizophrenic, narcissistic, and logically dissonant.

Declaring all things to have a purpose is pretty easy for the people sitting in the cheap seats. I know, because I've sat there myself, hurling useless clichés at the people in the arena below. Down in the trenches where the limbs are flying and there's blood everywhere, a Master Plan or someone's Greater Purpose doesn't do anything to stop the endless needles and the terror. You just want to the war to end so you can go home. You didn't volunteer anyway, you were drafted. Up in the cheap seats we can pontificate and theologize about higher purposes and belief to sound spiritual or wise, but after seeing so much suffering and cruelty, I just don't want to think about it anymore. At the expense of sounding un-spiritual, I think the fantasy that there's a Greater Good to come from all the suffering does little more than make us feel better about other people's tragedy. I've seen too much death and pain to make any substantial contribution to that conversation either, I guess, but the last thing I want to be guilty of is spiritualizing all of it so I can appear Godly or mature.

The irony would be amusing if it wasn't so sad; twenty-two people die in the U.S. every single day, waiting for an organ that never came. Others die because they waited so long that by the time they got one, they've gone into kidney failure, have life-threatening diabetes, atrophy, or have suffered strokes. Yet, the demographic that simultaneously offers up these spiritual platitudes also fights against and demonizes Universal Healthcare and donates the *least* number of organs on a yearly basis. Guess where the lion's share of donated organs come from?

Drug overdoses.

The way I see it, at least the junkie did something right in death, better than those who shuffle off this mortal coil with all of their parts, leaving seven people to die on their way to a heavenly reward. I know that makes me harsh and judgmental, but it's really damn hard to be nice about it when you're standing over a pile of dead friends. Needlessly.

Organ donation isn't a tricky thing. There are no theological conundrums. There isn't a single prohibition in any major world religion against organ donation. Then again, most people know their own theology about as well as I know the rules of basketball, but it seems like a cut-and-dried issue to me. There are no politics involved, no moral or ethical conflicts. Families tend not to donate their loved one's organs in their grief. Grief is an emotion, albeit the strongest emotion of all, after love for most. I hope I never have to make such a decision, but in this, and *so many other things*, American people have to start looking beyond the fog of emotion for just the briefest of moments to what is practical, to what is right. I hope that day comes. Because in the time it will take you to read the next two chapters of this book, a dozen more people have probably died waiting.

That's my pitch for organ donation, no extra charge. As for how to deal with the rising body count of the TAH club of which I'm the only remaining member, all I know to do is write a song about it.

Chapter 21

No Going Home

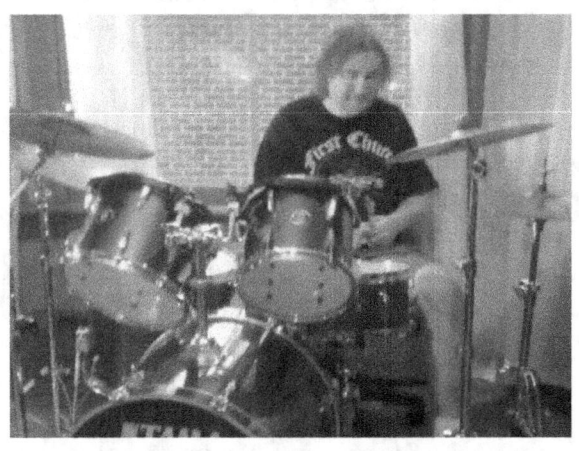

Remember a place, where everything fit?
Back in a time, when I knew where to sit
Sometimes I just run away, to clear my mind,
I knew that it wasn't forever, but at least it was mine

(Then the hurricane came)
Like a sledgehammer to a hovel,
and the mud washed it all away
I'll just bury it like bone-man with a shovel
And pretend I don't feel the pain
There's no going home

I had a face, that could stand up to them all
Now it falters and it creases, and I feel so small

*It was just a fantasy, nothing more than a dream
That it'd all be waiting for me, that they'd all know what I mean*

*Now that road just winds away
The path's overgrown and I feel like I've lost my way*

❝*How do you pick up the threads of an old life? How do you go on, when in your heart you begin to understand... there is no going back? There are some things that time cannot mend. Some hurts that go too deep, that have taken hold."* - J.R.R. Tolkien

Frodo Baggins struggles to understand why, after saving the world, after kings and nations have bowed before him, after defeating the impossible evil of Sauron, resisting the lure of the One Ring, and surviving the living death of Mordor, he finds himself. . . lost. He's sad, restless, and unfulfilled. Where there should be great relief and joy, he feels only grief, loss, and regret. The wound he sustained on Roundtop at the hands of the Witch King still causes him pain and will for the rest of his life. Yet, he's a considerably young Hobbit and has most of his life yet before him. Everything is backwards and upside down, and the simple pleasures of his home and life in the Shire for which he longed so deeply, leave him empty and restless.

This is how many stories end for characters of great literature who have been to places no one can imagine, seen things they can never really express, felt things that can't be articulated with adjectives. Jonah after his successful rescue of the Ninevites from God's wrath. Homer when he finally arrives home at the end of his Odyssey. Meg in A Wrinkle in Time. Bruce Wayne, Don Quixote, the list goes on.

Normal life is alien to me now. There is no nurse to call when I wake up. I can eat whenever I want. I can use the bathroom like a normal person without a urinal or tracking my input and output over a twelve-hour period. I can drive anywhere I want to. The grocery store. Restaurants. The park. I can buy most any food I crave. I can choose how to spend my time - no longer limited by my laptop and interacting with the handful of people on the unit that day.

I'm told there's something called "adjustment disorder," when a person has been forced to adhere to a schedule and restrained to a single environment for a length of time. It was best illustrated in the Stephen King book (and movie) The Shawhshank Redemption when the old gangster-turned-librarian, Brooks, is finally released from prison. The old man went in as a teenager and can't adjust to life on the outside. Everything confuses and overwhelms him. He eventually carves the simple epitaph "Brooks was here," in the rafter of his apartment where he hangs himself.

I spend a great deal of time doing nothing, or nothing that amounts to anything, simply because there's too much to choose from. The boys have learned a lot of independence in their school work and need me far less than they did when they were younger. Yet, I sporadically try to inject unwanted and unneeded projects and activities into the mix. Some days I poke around with recording sloppy demos of songs, scribble around on presentations for Gift of Life, cook a bit, play drums, and half-heartedly begin some project that needs to be finished at the house. Brian or Marc Gecker's invitations to join them for lunch are welcome interruptions.

Lost, in a word. Am I still a musician? Can I still call myself that? Am I a writer, or am I ready to abandon that? After five near misses with my two novels, I'm frustrated and feel paralyzed when it comes to pursuing agents, and I feel rejected by everyone and everything right now, legitimate or not. Why make it worse? I can't muster the interest to cook, and food still doesn't taste right. I've always been and remain inept at repair projects, and Christie's got to be tired of me leaving half-finished paint and patch jobs all over the house.

The hardest thing, the thing that I don't think I'll ever adjust to, is the way time has moved on here without me. The boys have grown up, and not just since I've been in the hospital. I've been checked out since before the TAH, what with the constant swans caths and hospitalizations, the ER visits for A-Fib, the pain meds that left me in a stupor on the couch the majority of the time. They're too old for the things we did when I was still moderately active, and Rich especially, as all teenagers, has reached a point where time with friends supersedes time with dad. Brennan, not so much, but he's slowly getting there. Where we used to connect over board games, watching TV, eating out, cooking together, or just going to the park, they only do those things now because they know I don't know what else to do with them. And I hate that they feel forced to patronize me.

It's like meeting that old friend that you've longed to catch up with so badly only to discover that so much time has passed, so much life and has come and gone, and experiences so changed you that you'll never truly know one another again, and that neither of you fit into the other's life as it is now. I know this isn't the case; my relationship with the boys will recover even from this. I just can't figure out how to adjust to the time lapse. I feel awkward and out of place with them, which only makes it worse.

I devote time to various groups, the HCMA, Gift of Life, and I try to volunteer at the hospital. Some of this is successful for a time. While Lisa, the founder of the HCMA, is recovering from heart transplant herself, I make her weekly phone calls to patients. I'm hesitant to say a word about my transplant; HCMers don't really associate the two things and I worry my assurances that there's hardly ever a need to transplant for HCM does little good, particularly as it's public knowledge that Lisa herself has now been transplanted. Eventually, she returns to work and I'm again searching for my place in this strange new life.

Gift of Life is the obvious place for a transplant patient to go, to do good, share their story, encourage people to become organ donors. Christie and I spend time in Philly at the Gift of Life family house and get to know some of the people in the organization. Maybe it's where I fit in. But my few opportunities to speak leave me frustrated. There's so little time and so much to say. How do you explain what's happened to your family, all the moving and false starts, all the changes, the four years of hospitalizations, the swans caths, the TAH, Perry, living on the HVI, the transplant, the rejections, the recovery...in five or ten minutes? It usually amounts to me racing to cram even a few of those in, always mentioning Perry (the part I refuse to leave out), and feeling like I've said little more than, "So, uh, I got transplanted, and uh, you should all be organ donors. Duh."

On a rainy day in October of 2016, I drag the boys to a game-con in a small hotel in Harrisburg. The event is sponsored by something called The Bodhana Group, and this is their annual fundraiser. We have a blast, but more importantly, learn that the group is a non-profit that uses RPG's and board gaming as adjunct therapy for kids with social adversities, learning handicaps, people in retirement centers, and dozens of other applications. I spend a lot of time talking with Jack Berkenstock, the executive director. He's a sharp-witted, artsy guy, dressed like a mid-90's British beatnik, and so full of energy, I feel hyperactive just being around him. He seems like part of my tribe. We strike upon an idea - how about using gaming to help people in long term care units in hospitals? What about kids in the cancer wards? Can it be done? Of course it can. Playing games is what helped us to pass long hours in waiting rooms and visits. It's how we got to know Perry, and he looked forward to playing every time we went to visit him. It's so obvious when I stop and think about it. I plan to use my contacts at Hershey to see what we can do.

Maybe this will turn into something. The HVI management seems increasingly reluctant to communicate and work with post-transplant patients to improve care on the unit, or to even make patients aware of our existence in case they want someone to talk to. Brian, Mudge, and I drop by as often as we can, but time is passing, and we know fewer and fewer nurses. We're starting to feel like strangers in a place that we once thought of as a home. This frustrates me and causes self-doubt as well. Is it me? Did I do something wrong?

After spending days in training, obtaining security clearances, background checks, blood draws, and jumping through various other hoops, my application to volunteer anywhere else in the hospital is rejected based on my prohibition from taking the Pertussis vaccine. It's one of the very few vaccines that contains a live virus, and it would be deadly for me to get the immunization. Understandably, this makes it dangerous for me to be around patients, as well as dangerous for them. Still, it feels like one more rejection, one more place where I don't fit in.

Perry was right. This is the hardest part. The drugs are making it worse by playing tricks on my brain but it's impossible to separate what's in my head from what's reality. Regardless, I'm determined to explore all avenues. There must be somewhere I should be, something I should be doing to make a difference. I didn't go through all of this to sit at home, slop my way through home renovations, and cook dinner every once in a while. Not being active is like a poison inside me. I've never been able to sit still and consume. I want to interact and produce. I need to.

In January of 2017, by biopsy shows no rejection, but the dreaded CMV virus that resides in the hearts of about 50% of the population – including my donor's - rears its ugly head while I'm over-immunosuppressed over the holidays. We knew it was there, but early medications should have made it a non-issue. This means going back on even more immunosuppression, to the point that I become neutropenic - a walking virus and germ magnet - and have to quarantine myself at home for three months. If I was having trouble finding my place in this new life, the next few months make me begin to doubt that I belonged anywhere at all. It becomes the darkest road I've travelled so far.

Chapter 22

All Go Down

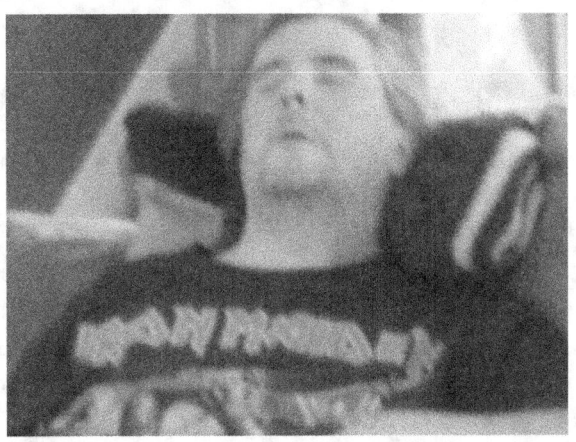

If I'm bitter, who's to blame
If I'm angry all the time, why should I stay
You don't know the faces, you don't know the names
You don't know the melting of the flesh underneath the flame
Sometimes...there's nothing to do,
sometimes...you got to wear the shoes

And we would all down together
And my guilt would float away like a feather
We would all go down,
leave the safety of the beach and drown
All go down together

If I'm falling apart, I'll blame the poison,
If I'm lashing out, I'll blame the bruises and the blood and-
Raise a glass to all the wounded, the broken and the dead
Raise a gun to still the black parade
marching through my head
Sometimes, there's nothing you can do,
sometimes, you've got to walk in the shoes

Stumbling over landmines, trying to get back home
Just can't find a passage through the spit, the blood,
and splintered bones

The water trickles across the basement floor from the torrential rain outside. We've become accustomed to the minor flooding of basements in this part of the country. It's February 2017 and the space heater at my feet warms the little cave I've made for myself to keep me from freezing. I'm surrounding by recording equipment, a drum set and various guitars in my dark little hideout, but it's too loud to actually make serious recordings down here because of the constant noise of the water heater and the clicking of the dog's claws on the hardwood floor above. I've been recording demos for what I hope will be a companion to this book I've been writing since about September. But I don't feel like recording anything much today. I crank on my Carvin amp and start pounding out the angriest chords I know over and over on my Washburn. Being a drummer at heart, I'm extremely hard on guitar strings because of the rhythmic aggressiveness that carries over from hitting things to express myself. The same three chords in various succession. It's the only thing that will come out of me and it's not pretty. It becomes this song - All Go Down.

I don't sleep at night anymore. Mainly, I lay with my eyes closed, thinking of Bentonville, again. Of the library and gym with Brennan, and volunteering at Rich's school. Of the homeschool group we joined that year, the friends we made. I think of how happy I was, writing a book, finally free from the self-imposed entanglement of ministry. Things were really simple then, and I've worked my mind into a corner; this nostalgia feels like the only solace from the side-effects of the Prograf, the sporadic nightmares, and constant sense of grief and loss that's spiraling out of control. I've stopped cooking and haven't looked at Facebook in a few weeks. I only check to make sure no one is desperately trying to message me about something.

But why would they? What obligations do I really have to anyone? What all-important Thing am I part of that would necessitate anyone needing my attention for anything? I'm trapped here, in my basement hideaway, where I won't yell at my kids, and take my frustrations out on Christie. They've been through enough. Their sacrifice and long-suffering were supposed to all pay off on the other side of transplant. I don't think it has.

With the emergence of this CMV, revealed at my last biopsy in January, has come a deadly serious susceptibility to germs and bacteria. I've been instructed not to answer the door or even drive thru a fast food window, for fear that I may contract something from someone. My immune-system has to take one for the team if the CMV virus is to be put down. The first week of the new year, I'd hesitantly ventured into a men's barbershop chorus (the same group from which came the quartet that sang to me in the cath lab recovery on Valentine's day all the way back in 2014). I was getting my voice back in shape after four years of nothing but home studio singing, and the camaraderie was a shot in the arm. I've had to quit that now, as well as drop several commitments with Gift of Life and The Bodhana Group. All of these represented new roads, new beginnings, new relationships. I'd barely begun to get acclimated, only to now abruptly disappear for three months. Of course, everyone understands, but it likely did nothing to help establish my dependability or consistency with anyone. And when you're the new guy, it's assumed that this is just how you are. Flaky. Why bother doing anything if I'm just going to end up being forced to quit every time some new, unexpected problem appears? What's the point?

Is it the meds? Everything finally catching up with me? This isn't the life I imagined at the end of all this. My kid's lives have moved on without me, and I feel like a stranger no matter where I am. The familiar faces that I wish were near - Perry, my old bandmates, our Arkansas homeschool friends, may as well be on another planet. As much as I've tried to hold on to my identity as a songwriter and musician, I play nowhere, I play with no one. I sit in a basement writing angry songs about death and sickness that no one will ever want to hear. It feels like that part of myself is dying, slipping away beyond my grasp. Publishing agents have flirted with and dumped me so many times by now that I don't care if I ever successfully sell a book. Let the whole industry burn and stoke the fires with pop-culture stupidity like Twilight and James Patterson. Let Miley Cyrus and Pitbull rule the airwaves. Tear it all down.

What I do have is a house that's been in disrepair since we bought it, and even more so because there's been no time or money for the necessary upkeep. What projects I force myself to start, usually end in abject frustration and even tears. I've never been good at that type of stuff. My dad has astonishing talent with wood. He and my brother Darrell have the enviable gift of knowing intuitively how to build or fix things on the spot. So does my father-in-law and Christie, which explains where Rich gets it from. Brennan and I typically watch while our minds wander into the lands of fantasy, science fiction, or music. I've never had an interest in or knack for things like hanging drywall, painting, electrical work, home repair, plumbing or anything remotely related to any of that. I can build a computer, chart music, write anything you challenge me to, and even draw a bit. I play four instruments, write songs, sing, perform, speak, write, and have some cosmic grasp on Latin and Middle-Eastern languages. If a toilet won't stop running, I'm more likely to come with a novella or a song about it than to know how to fix it. Regardless of the fact that the perpetually running toilet is a phenomenon that we all encounter over and over again in our lives. I'm pretty sure we'll all survive without another song or story.

My lack of skill and knowledge is amplified by the minute as I stalk around the house like a caged animal. The bannister needs to be replaced. The back fence needs to be weather-proofed before another winter. There's a water spot on the kitchen ceiling. We need to hang fans and reconfigure lighting. The floors need to be refinished - a job I actually know how to do but have been sternly warned against by the transplant team because sanding old floors stirs up dust. Until the modern era, stain was colored using organic materials - in other words, pig's blood - that carry pathogens that could be deadly for me to inhale.

How is this any different from life with HCM? Isolated, diminished, overwhelmed with things that need to be done, but unable to do them. I've turned into an ogre, living in my cave, surrounded by drums, guitars, and microphones that I don't want to look at any more, much less use.

Is it my ego? So many people checked on and worried about me for so long, and now the storm has passed, leaving me here. I'm not sick anymore, not really. I have the energy and the physical strength to do most anything, but this quarantine has taken away any opportunity beyond what I had when I lived in the hospital. I should have never gone through with the transplant, dragged my family through all of this, just for me to be sullen and lost. I can only think of the things I'll never get back. The boy's childhoods, my youth with my wife, my chance to have a career, to play music, to work and be financially stable, to build lasting friendships that are safe from the predation of distance and time. And I feel as trapped as if I had died and were stuck in a casket, buried in the ground.

Against doctor's orders I finally see a therapist a few times, wearing a mask and avoiding the waiting room by lingering outside in the cold until he comes to get me.

"It's the same thing we see in soldiers who've been in action," he tells me.

"I'm not a soldier." I'm appalled to be compared to one. I didn't volunteer to defend anyone with my life.

"Was your life in constant danger?" he asks causally.

"Yeah, but it's not like anyone was trying to purposely kill me. That was just biology."

"Did people around you die from the same threat you were under?"

This one's harder to get around.

"Well...yeah."

"Did you at any time think you weren't going to survive?"

Of course. "I was determined to, but the numbers weren't on my side."

"And you were gone from your normal life, your family for more than a few weeks." He leans forward in his chair. "Any one of these conditions puts a normal person's body into a fight or flight mode. Your body manufactures chemicals that cause chain reactions throughout your system, but they also cause things to happen in your brain. It alters the way you process things. That's why it's called POST-traumatic stress disorder. It doesn't affect you until those conditions change. Then you react.

"The other thing is the survivor's guilt. Most transplanted people have this over their donor. You don't seem to. What you do have is an entirely disproportionate amount of survivor's guilt over fellow patients that didn't make it. You're essentially the last man standing. You can't celebrate surviving because the people you want to celebrate that with are gone."

There may be something to all this psychology stuff, I think.

"You're not sliding back into life at home because you can't adjust. Reality doesn't reflect your expectations. But I don't think you need me to tell you any of this because you're not stupid."

"I don't want to be put on more meds," I say. I'm desperate not to. I can barely tolerate the ones I'm on now.

"I'm not going to give you any. It seems to me that you're not finished grieving your friends, but you will be, in your own time. You're also ready to do a million things because you feel better than ever. But your family is exhausted. Watching TV is a waste of time to you, but to them it's recovery. There's no running back and forth to the hospital and worrying about you. They're still defusing, and you have to give them the time they need to do that."

"That's it?" Nothing I don't know but hearing it from someone else somehow makes it okay to admit I'm fighting with this stuff.

The nightmares are the worst part of it. I can't tell who these recurring characters are; some bizarre Frankenstein combination of Perry and Blake, or Jamie and Dot, or James and Perry. Emaciated, blood shot eyes, pale, and angry, shouting names and unformed words at me from all sides. They disappear when I try to look directly at them, but I know the voice. My subconscious isn't very subtle, so none of this bears dream interpretation or a psychological translation.

I'm baffled by my inability to deal with all of this on my own. I've got a fairly large tool kit filled with most of what I need to help others through such things. During my years in ministry, I've been threatened, slandered, lied to and about, rejected, neglected, publicly mocked, thrown out of places, spit on, and embezzled from. Why now, at this point, when I should be looking forward, do I not have the tools I need to work past these things? There is no shortage of people telling me that I shouldn't be hung up on them, over it, that I should be able to let these things go. Empathy from some quarters, but Christie's really the only one who knows the extent of the struggle I'm having and why. The boys see it, but can I really expect them to understand why I'm a listless mess after having survived everything else?

Like anything else in life, you had to be there. I wonder a lot if it makes me a bad person to wish that the people in my life could, just for a few minutes, experience the isolation, the fear of watching everyone go down around you. Or just briefly, the pain of a swans cath or TAH site change or the panic that tries to overtake your good sense when your brain starts screaming, "You didn't even have a heart! What were you? Were you even human?" I don't know where to put any of this. I don't have boxes for any of it, let alone a shelf to put them on, and I have no idea how I would begin to define or label any of it.

In retrospect, it was a lot of self-pity and too much introspection, but that's what happens when you jack someone up on steroids and lock them away for three months. I don't think it would have been so bad, except to my mind, I'd already been locked away to some degree for eighteen years, the last five months of that quite literally. I eventually come to believe that this is what life is like at the end of my journey. I have no choice but to change my expectations and adjust to the opposite of my former circumstance; for a long time, I was sick, but free. Now I'm well, but a captive.

Chapter 23

Turn

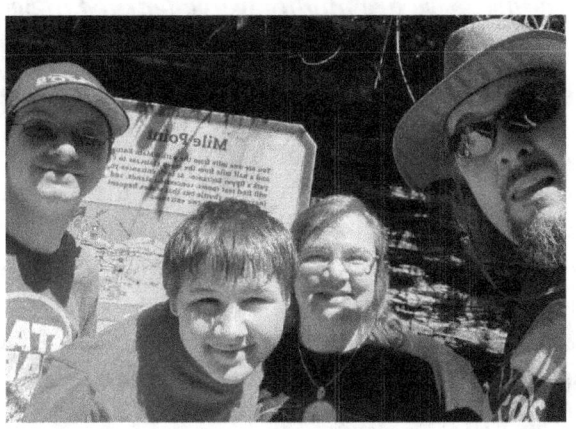

All these dark places, from which we can't escape
Memories and regret, fill me with purpose, fill me with rage
The brightest light still casts shadows, murderous and dark
Holding on to you and me, letting go of what we've lost

And we turn, remember who we are
And we turn, we've made it this far

Long overdue, this valley is treacherous, he tried to tell us
The other side of the sun,
but the storms rage, even under this umbrella
The brightest light hurts my eyes,
bleaches my skin, leaves me thirsty

The mountain behind, but we've learned, what will be will be

And we turn, remember who we are
And we turn, we've made it this far

Turning corners, turning pages, turn around
Lay to rest the sickness, that kept me buried in the ground
Let go the lifeline, lose a burden, forsake the lost and found
Lay aside another tie that kept me bound, and turn around

And we turn – we are mighty we've learned to be brave
And we turn – one with the beauty one with the pain

The sound of water again, but not of a leaky basement. It laps against the side of a kayak. Rich sits in front, watchfully nervous and trying to steer the best he can as we float out toward the center of the lake. It's my first time in a kayak, my first time to hold a paddle in my hands, to be honest. Outside of a paddle boat, I've never been responsible for myself on a large body of water. It's invigorating, to be in danger of capsizing; a small danger over which I have some modicum of control. I push all that out of my mind and try to soak in the breeze, the sun, the sound of the water. "Being mindful" everyone calls it now. I only know that a year ago, I couldn't have dreamed that I'd be in the middle of a lake in a kayak, with no tubes or wires attached, showered, fed, and nearly six hours away from my transplant team or hospital. My only attachment to all of that are the meds sitting in my pack on the shore. My hair has grown out again, and the wind blows through it, sending a chill down my back. I don't mind the heat and cold so much anymore. I consider the unpredictable weather a joy in comparison to the steadily maintained seventy-two-degree room that was my world back then. The breeze may blow us too far from shore but realize I can paddle back with my full strength if need be.

  We've spent three days in Bath, New York. It's the first true vacation the boys can remember that wasn't centered around an Echo or appointment. Neither was it a rushed trip to Arkansas where we strain and stress to see our families without ever seeming to have enough time. We've stayed up late playing our favorite games and slept in late in our little log cabin, safe from the beeps and blats of our phones due to the terrible cell reception. We've explored during the day. The Corning glass factory yesterday. Finger Lakes today. Maybe a state park for some hiking tomorrow. Christie and I rode bikes around the campsite before dinner yesterday too. I've been riding with Marc Gecker a few times a week. I'm up to a mile and a half so far. My muscles are finally sore from exercise instead of atrophy. No biopsies for another six months. My team doesn't know or care where I am, which should be unsettling, after being tied to them at the wrist for nearly three years - and my Tuft's team for a year before that. I could get used to this.

***

Back home, Joe is helping me with my bow tie. I'm in a tux for the first time since my wedding. I always stand next to old Joe in the front row when our barbershop chorus sings, and we've become fast friends he and I; the heavy metal drummer and the eighty-something small engine pilot. He keeps me moving and in key. It's our annual "pay the rent" show and Christie and the boys are there in the back, smiling as we rip through renditions of Delta Dawn, Roger Miller's King of the Road, and a few Sinatra tunes, that bring out the ham in both Joe and me. Four of the guys on the platform came to sing for me on a Valentine's Day back in 2014 but they have no idea of all that's transpired since then. I promised them I'd be singing with them one day. I'm the youngest in the group, discounting the leader's grandson, and they remind me that you don't have to die before you get old.

When the gig is finished, I introduce Christie and the boys around to everyone; Carl and his wife, who tell us stories of the blackouts on the Baltimore shore during the Nazi naval scares during the War. Richard scoffs about soldiers returning from Afghanistan with PTSD. "I shot a dozen north Koreans. Haven't lost a night of sleep. Bastards were trying to kill me, so I killed 'em right back." I just roll my eyes and laugh. He shrugs and shuffles off to get more desert from the buffet. They all comment on how polite and articulate the boys are. No one here really knows our story, and we don't tell it unless asked. I don't really care if they ever know. It's enough just to be in a room with people living normal lives.

***

The woman pushes the elevator button, then sighs.

"I pushed the wrong floor," she tells Brennan and me. We're the only other people on board. We're coming up from seeing Christie down in Radiology.

"No problem," I say, "we're not in a hurry."

"I've been here since Sunday night," she says wearily. This elicits sympathetic nods from both of us. "People just don't understand – it all starts to blur together."

She looks up at the numbers and Brennan and I share a small grin. It's only Monday afternoon. I recall again the scene at the end of Tolkien's Return of the King where the four Hobbits share a drink at the Old Red Dragon. Life swirls on around them, people busy with their lives as the four of them just sit and take it in. No one knows they all nearly died saving Middle-Earth. They lift their glasses, give each other a knowing look, and enjoy the moment. We find ourselves in these moments more and more often.

***

I pause and look back at the massive, mid-20's, three story house in which I've spent the last three days. Jack, the director of The Bodhana Group, recommended me to go through the training to be a volunteer at Olivia's House, a non-profit (who graciously waived the typically expensive training fee for me). They run programs for children and teens who have lost loved ones in violent deaths and Bodhana runs games for these groups as adjunct therapy; I'll be joining Jack in the future in that endeavor. I've heard horror stories over the last three days, but also stories of hope. The meetings are over, and everyone has left, so I'm walking across the vacant lot next door to my parking spot in the rear, and the weight of change comes over me. It's getting dark, and this is a bad neighborhood, but I sit with my back to a smelly dumpster and stare up at the windows of Olivia's House. How did I end up here? I've driven myself crazy trying to find ways to help on the HVI, to work with Gift of Life, but it was all a terrible fit. Here, with The Bodhana Group and these Olivia House volunteers, is the first time I've felt...home. I can't be involved yet. It's an hour from home and the groups meet on a difficult night of the week. The Room 1170 project is consuming every spare second of my time. But something stirs in me and I know I'll be back here, that this place is in my future one way or another. I tear up a little, a near-daily habit of mine since the transplant. More often than not these days, it's either the small amount of Prednisone in my system, or tears of happiness, rather than grief. The winds of change blowing, I can tell. I remember the Russ Taff song that's been rattling around in my head for about three decades now:

"Hunger is no stranger, I've sat with him before,
And everything I've done has not been good.
But as I've learned to make my stand, I've had to learn to fall
And maybe I have seen more than I should...
The hands of time go round and round,
they don't slow down when you lose your way
At every turn, the things you learn, you wear them proud
like you wear your name
And as you go on down that road,
don't let the dust get in your eyes...
It blows in the wind of change..."

Conversations from Room 1170

(The Winds of Change – Russ Taff)

***

"Your infusion is finished, want me to turn it off?" I ask Craig. He's nineteen, lanky but athletic, tell-tale baldness of cancer treatment. We met an hour ago, but conversation comes easily once I tell him I'm post-transplant.

"Sure," he says. I notice one of the interns frown when I reach over and hit the "finish" button on Craig's own Dr. Doo-daa. We're talking about hospital food over a game of King Domino. The Bodhana Group is sponsoring a game day at the John Hopkins Children's hospital. Though I'm usually Jack's shadow at Bodhana events, watching and learning, here, it's just me and Emma, another intern who volunteers with our group. Baltimore was an hour and a half drive this morning, but I'll drive twice as far to sit in a room with long-term care patients. I'd pay money to do it.

When I was a pastor, I'd beg my assistant, Richard Douglas, to do it for me. I was terrible – awkward, foot in mouth, fidgety. Rich is a natural and seems to float in cloud of peace and comfort in that setting, so I always delegated it to him.

More and more, I feel drawn to be with sick people. Not to bring them sage wisdom, or inspiration, or even company. I'm most comfortable in my own skin around them, and they seem comfortable with me, either playing games, talking, or just sitting in silence.

Craig and I share a shorthand that eludes the nurses and interns who wander by.

"How long this time?" I ask. Obviously, it's not his first – his hairlessness tells me that.

"Ten weeks for the program, but only two days at a time. This is my second round." He's supposed to be in college on a basketball scholarship. Arrested development. Sounds familiar.

"Everything else goes on hold. Sucks," I say, taking the last tile.

"I don't think about the stretch. There's just the first day and the last day."

Don't I know it.

"Whoa, Ryan!" I jump up and grab the five-year old's Dr. Doo-da and pull it closer to the giant Connect Four he's jumping around in front of. "Be careful, buddy, you're gonna pull your lines too far." He nods distractedly and goes back to jumping up to insert a big checker in one of the slots.

"Ryan freaks most volunteers out," one of the nurses tells me later, while we're boxing up games. "They've never seen a toddler with an IV and PICC line."

"Eh, he's just like any other kid. I had to guard the Dippin' Dots machine after his fourth one. I always assume diabetes, just to be safe." I learn later Ryan's actually under-going pre-treatments for a bone marrow transplant.

"It's good for the parents when visitors are comfortable around the kids. Some people just can't handle it," she says. "I think it's a gift to be able to deal with medical stuff, especially when it comes to children."

I don't tell her about my transplant, just nod and smile. It's the third time I've been to John Hopkins for one thing or another. The military kid from Arkansas, the heavy metal drummer who was sitting in his own sterile room less than two years ago, wondering if a world still existed outside, beyond the four walls. All I wanted to do was leave. Now, places like this feel like a home away from home. But it's not because of the smells, the sterility, the lab coats, and IV poles. It's because of the people who live here know. They know, unlike anyone else can ever know, and none of us have to explain it to each other. There's an immense comfort in that, on both sides, I think.

***

It's Organ Donor month, and Gift of Life has invited me to spend the afternoon in the surgical break room meeting people on the teams. They rarely if ever get to see the results of their work in the flesh. The surgeon follows up on the floor – I see Dr. Soleimani around the hospital about once a month now. But the rest of the team does their job, gets 'em in, gets 'em out, and never really knows how things turn out. I'd never thought about it before.

"I've held your heart in my hand," one woman tells me. "I remember you, because I also held your TAH when he took it out. Your hair's gotten long."

She can't talk for long – I don't even get her name, and I'm not allowed to take a picture. She grabs a piece of the cake we've brought, gives me a big bear hug and she's off again, back to the OR. There was a heart transplant last night and as always, word gets around quick, but today it's someone else, with some other crisis. About thirty people pop in and out over the rest of the day, and I meet about four people who were in at least one of my surgeries. Cal, another transplant buddy who's twenty-seven years out, gives me a pep talk about staying in shape. He avoids the cake and we get a rare picture together. I hope I make it to twenty-seven years. Right now, I'm just glad I got to be here today.

***

I sit at my friend Marc's kitchen table, coffee between us.

"You'll never guess who I saw last night," he says. "Joy!" He doesn't wait for me to answer.

"THE Joy?" I ask. I've heard stories. Marc is approaching seventy and he loves to tell stories about his wild youth as a doctoral program dropout who grew his hair, hitchhiked through Europe, and "smoked more weed than Willie Nelson."

"Ellen," says Marc, "is the love of my life. Joy was the love of my youth." I often live vicariously through Marc as he remembers the 60's; I always say I was born fifteen years too late. To have been a teen when Hendrix, The Beatles, Joplin, Zeppelin, The Who, and all the others were in their hey-day - it seems like a fantasy world that people lived in. "Imagine it," he tells me, "you're just driving down the road and the DJ comes on and says, here's a brand new one from the Rolling Stones, and stay tuned, next up, the first single from the new Cream album." How can I be so nostalgic for a time period I never even experienced?

"We were at a meeting for Ellen's business," he goes on, "and there she was - she got up to speak and I couldn't believe it! I haven't seen her for nearly fifty years." The two of them had quite the adventures, sometimes on the wrong side of the local police, went through primal therapy together ("an abysmal failure," says Marc), and eventually grew apart.

"What did you say to her?" I asked.

"Nothing. I didn't talk to her. Really wish I hadn't seen her."

This puzzles me. He's never uttered an angry word toward anyone that I can remember and talks about Joy with great melancholy and happiness.

"Yeah, okay," I say. "Wait, no. You have to explain that to me. As usual."

"Because I wanted to remember her as she was, when we were young, reckless kids, not as a matronly older woman."

As someone who goes to great lengths to stay connected to people, even long after any vestiges of a relationship have withered away, this seems Anathema to me. He knows me well enough now to know my, "Marc, you're being senile" look.

He takes a sip and carefully places his mug down. "I don't hold onto things or people," he says patiently. "Me and Joy - that was a moment in time. I've closed that box and tucked it away in my memory to pull out from time to time if I want. There are no more chapters to write. I'm married to Ellen, and Joy's moved on. So much time has passed - why would I try to resurrect a relationship that I remember fondly and possibly ruin that for both of us? We said goodbye, knowing we might never see each other again, and that was that. I want to cherish what it was, not what it might be now - it can't be the same, and I'm happy with my memories."

And there it is. Just like that. The solution.

The bulk of my self-torture over these months and years has nothing to do with the way things are now. They have to do with things not being the way they were then. My marriage was interrupted in its first decade by HCM. My boy's childhoods interrupted by acute heart failure. My aspirations interrupted by chronic heart failure. So much loss, more than I feel I can bear to think about at times. But in the midst, memories. Small pieces of time, little moments, phases, that I've tucked away in some vain hope that I'll feel that way again, that life will bring me the same joys that it did at those times. How many nights have I fallen asleep with a film of the boys digging in the sandbox in Bentonville playing in my mind? Or the four of us walking around the block with Nanouq, them riding ahead in the motorized yellow truck? Me and Christie snuggled on the couch watching Friends on VHS until three in the morning and eating ice-cream with Robin? All of it was interrupted by this disease, cut short.

But life is a series of interruptions. My problem is that I don't think I'll ever have the peace and contentment that I had before. And that frightens and frustrates me.

And here is the solution.

Rob Thomas of Matchbox 20 wrote a song called *These Small Hours* for the Disney movie Meet the Robinsons. Neither did well commercially, but the song is one of my favorites:

"Our lives are made, in these small hours,
These little moments, these twists and turns of fate
Life slips away, but these small hours,
These small hours will remain,
And all of my regret, just falls away somehow
But I will not forget, the way it feels right now"

(These Small Hours – Rob Thomas)

When is the right time to close the door on something you'll never get back? How long before I can relegate those cherished times and feelings to a closed box to be put on the shelf and only opened to remember, rather than to mourn?

I'm visibly disturbed and Marc can tell.

"You okay?" he asks.

"No," I whisper, wiping away a fugitive tear. "I'm rattled. How can you just...put it in a box? What if it could be a good thing? What if she's married now and you and Ellen could be friends with her and her husband? How do you know it might not be better?"

"Is it ever really better? I can't remember anything ever living up to the spontaneous original. There's only one first time for everything. You have to know when to be satisfied, otherwise you're always trying to recapture old glory. There's plenty of new glory to be had, you just have to keep moving."

I drive home the long way again that morning, out by the VA hospital where the trees are plentiful. I don't listen to music, pull into a space for the walking park down from our house. And then it comes.

The director of Olivia's House told me that we're all in a constant state of loss. Loss of a job, loss of a favorite TV show, loss of a potential friendship. To be human is to lose things. The more important the thing we lose, the more alarmed we are over losing small things, like our keys or wallet.

I don't know what to call the thing that came pouring out of me that morning. It was primal, and animalistic. I screamed and wept and pounded the steering wheel for a good ten minutes. Thank God no one saw me, they would have called the police or the guys in the white coats. I sobbed until my throat ached.

I couldn't cry when I had the TAH - the crunching of stomach muscles ("vagaling down") caused the alarms to go crazy. No crying unless you wanted to announce to everyone that you were. It hurt too bad to cry after the transplant - though I did it a little - because of the scarring. Even through the depression of that spring, I didn't cry. I didn't have the energy.

She also told me that it's impossible to truly process loss until you mourn. When have I mourned? There's been no time. So many things to mourn, coming one on top of the other that I could barely think about them, much less mourn them. I think that's what I did that morning. Going all the way back to my late twenties, I mourned losing my bands, my business, my house, my musical career that was just taking off. I mourned losing the youth of my marriage to life and death troubles instead of enjoying the carefree days before parenthood. I mourned not being able to coach Rich's little league or soccer team, and not being able to teach Brennan how to ride a bike. I mourned myself, watching from a pool chair as other dads wrestled and tossed their kids around the swimming pool, and the ball field, and the yard. I mourned my isolation and loneliness while those around me carried on with life as usual while I felt guilty for not helping friends move, or showing up to play paintball, or for just not being able to do a single thing that didn't make me feel anti-social and apart.

And I mourned our family in Bentonville, the loss of our walks around the block, mine and Brennan's library, Rich's excitement when it was my day to be a Watchdog Dad. I mourned little Brennan, six years ago as he stood in the library foyer, clinging to Sue-Anne, the children's librarian, and sobbing as he said goodbye to her for the last time. And his tears five years later as we sat on the stoop outside again for a rare visit. The friends we made only to lose as we rambled around New England, scared to death that I was out of time, trying to counter the endless hours in waiting rooms with trips to museums and parks, desperately trying to do the best we could to make things normal and knowing we couldn't.

I cried for the relationships fallen by the wayside, the people who couldn't or wouldn't follow us through this, the failed communication, the lapse of time, the disconnect from so many things that were impossible to explain now that so much life has passed by.

I raged for my kids, trying to do schoolwork on laptops in waiting rooms while they knew someone was either cutting on me or jamming wires into my heart a few rooms over. For the time spent with people they didn't choose, in the back seats of cars, carried back and forth like so much luggage to see whatever was left of me for years at a time, only to return home to an empty house because Christie still had to work. And I raged for her, for the endless blocks of days without sleep that became her life during the TAH, and a career put on hold to the point of job termination because there was no time for required classes, and long overdue degrees. Her loss of freedom, choice, familiarity, and a spouse that could actually be a partner.

And I pounded my fist at whatever God or power could stand by and watch Perry, so full of life and wisdom, bleed to death while his mother and sisters looked on helplessly. Perry who'd not taken a free breath from the time he was seven years old. I mourned him too, and Jamie, and Dot, and Joe, and Blake, and James.

But the good parts started going on a shelf. Perry's pranks and Blake's bouncing energy. Dot's sardonic quips and Jamie's Eeyore complaints about the itchy TAH dressing. Christie and I at Universal Studios in Florida, long ago, and the night Rich was born, finally in the peace and quiet of a room with this impossible miracle asleep on my chest. The Thursday night gang and our Sunday night X-Files and Chinese food rituals with Robin, Leslie, Jason, Tiffany, and Spencer. Racing to get the floors cleaned at Holiday Inn so we could get home before one in the morning, and both hating and loving working for ourselves. Teaching the boys to eat crab legs in Boston and discovering Indian food in Connecticut. The look on Smitty's face when The Dreadnaughts or Ground Zero nailed a really hard song, whether there were ten or a hundred people in the crowd. Joking around with my brothers on holidays, and weekend trips down the mountain to see our parents. Nanouq, curled up by the back rug in the mornings when I made breakfast before taking Rich to school.

I could write a book about both - the mourning, and the boxes. I'm still holding some of the boxes because I can't quite put them on the shelf yet. There are still things to put in them but they won't quite fit yet. Soon.

The thing about organizing a closet and putting all the boxes where they belong is that you can't stand there staring at them forever. You may as well crawl inside and shut the door behind you. The world is over your shoulder, waiting. The boxes aren't going anywhere, and there's nothing to see in them that you haven't already seen. Life is moving on behind your back, and at some point, you have to close the closet door and turn around.

Chapter 24

Rest Assured

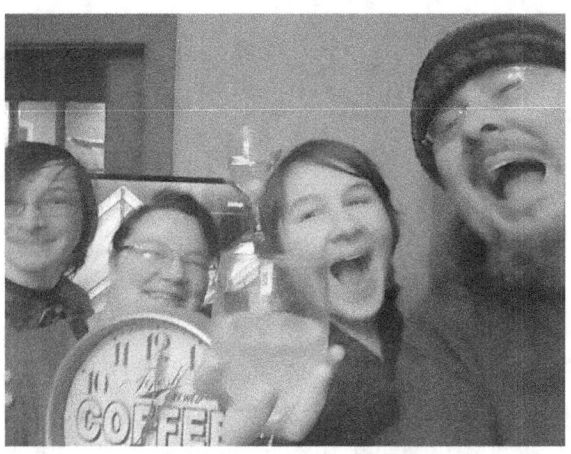

*(There must be some way out of here,
I keep singing to the break of day,
This darkness won't hold me down,
True love keep shining though, we're all going to find our way
To the top of the hill, if we can learn to be still
This gulf's too wide for anyone to cross alone
We're all gonna find a home, under the scorching sun
No more wasting time, 'cause the wind just blows…and blows)*

*Rest assured, time keeps moving on
Lay my head down where I belong
Where drunken fate has no more sting
Pain behind us, flight by Phoenix wing*

Conversations from Room 1170

Rest assured, time's on our side
No guilt, no pride, we've done our time
Whatever future we pursue
In search of peace long overdue

Our ever fire-escape, our ever home
To ease my mind, to mend my broken bones
Our ever bird's eye view, all that we can see
Whatever comes, we'll be ready...

Rest assured, time keeps moving on,
Time for me to wake up and face the dawn

It's a small whisper in my ear, just behind me, not loud enough for anyone else to hear.

"I need to do a skin assessment."

Larry.

I spin around and we hug one another fiercely. He's grown his beard out and he's leaving at three in the afternoon – way earlier than his old shift on the HVI. We're standing in the lobby, a piano and lap steel duo playing in the background where Shelba still performs every month or so.

We talk about the heat, the Kix concert he went to the other night, and Chuck, who's moved on to a new job too. Christie still sees him a lot downstairs at her new job in Radiology, but I'm not here as often as I used to be. Even though I still feel like I own the place, so much has changed. Float and travel nurses occupy the majority the stations on the HVI. The main thing that's changed is I don't even have to be here that much anymore. There was a time I didn't know how to function outside of the place. Now it just looks like a hospital to me, though there are lots of memories hidden away in boxes in the back of my mind. I'm learning to keep the closet door closed instead of ajar, so I can look at them when

I want to, instead of them always looming out at me. I'm successful about half the time.

I do the psychiatric thing with Dr. Hayes, new guy to the team, who's trying to help me work through some of the mess. Yes, I'm still having nightmares, but only every few weeks now. Yes, I'm trying to hurry up and finish this "Conversations from Room 1170" project because it's causing me to dwell on difficult things. Yes, I've talked to Sam (Perry's sister) lately. No, we actually didn't talk about Perry.

I talk to Brian on the way home. Hernia surgery next week. Mudge needs hip surgery but needs to lose weight. We're both worried about him. We share our aches and pains like old men.

"Do you ever get those sharp pains in your feet - like at the end of your toes?"

"Yeah...maybe a few times a week."

"Think it's the Cellcept?"

"Probably the Prograf. I gotta see a neurologist again

to see what's going on."

"I gotta call and see why they won't fill this Tramadol again. We doing lunch tomorrow?"

"Yeah, if I can. This hernia hurts like hell."

"I bet. This one at the base of my sternum is getting worse, but they can't really do anything about it."

"Oh well. Any day this side of the grass."

"Any day, this side of the grass, brother."

I get Brennan through an algebra lesson, throw some food in the crockpot, then sit down to pay bills and check on any new documents that have been added to the RPG I've been asked to direct for The Bodhana Group. The rest of the day is spent touching up guitar tracks and mixing for the album.

There are new things. Instead of begging favors from old friends, I meet a guitar player over the web who's adding all the lead guitars to the album. A brand-new designer is working on the book and album cover, and I'm forcing myself to relinquish some control. These unfamiliar creative relationships spark things in my brain and make me want to start a hundred other projects. But I have to finish this one.

The Bodhana RPG has breathed new life into our house. We spent weeks renovating the basement to make a meeting/game room for the team that will be creating this new world from nothing. It feels great to work on a project together, and on launch day, our house is filled once again with the sounds of laughter, new friends, new stories, and anticipation of new paths. The boys and I will be working on stories and art together, an unexpected surprise that makes me want to wrap up this book and album all the sooner.

Christie is back to school, working straight through to her master's degree, now that there's little fear of unexpected ER trips or last-minute admissions. Brennan is back to fencing, like he did in Springfield, and Rich is playing soccer again. Stitch and Blitzy, our two rescue dogs, are no Nanouq, but keep me either laughing or irritated enough to keep that box on the shelf. It's one that still makes me cry more than laugh when I open it up, but I've begun to leave it there more often and play with the new pups instead.

I've had a terrible bout of rejection after a med change at the end of 2017. One of my anti-rejection pills was causing migraines, so the docs switched me, but the dosage wasn't quite right. No damage done, but two familiar battles with Prednisone and a resulting sinus infection that lasted five months. I've despaired of ever being able to really get my voice back or play live music again. Maybe that's not who I am anymore. Maybe I'm the guy who writes RPG's for a non-profit and taxis the kids around. I'm a nurse's husband, a dog owner, and a board game enthusiast who at one time was going to conquer the world from behind a drum set, before a wasting disease found him.

In the process of grief, there's a step we call "acceptance." I think that's a crappy step. I will never accept that any of this was okay, or even meant to be. I won't accept the heavy price that my wife and boys had to pay for me to be alive. I won't accept that Perry was supposed to die, and I was supposed to live. I won't accept that story to soothe my guilt over my donor's death either.

I've chosen to change it from "acceptance" to "assimilation." I will always be a drummer, and I will always be a husband and father. The transplant did away with my disease, but I will always be an HCM patient, and I will identify with all the people who suffer from it. I will always be angry about Perry's and Jamie's deaths - to be otherwise is to say that it's okay, to normalize the shortage of organs and the indifference of a population in which the largest demographic of donors are drug users who have overdosed. While our religious country praises God for their new cars and their health, and comprise the smallest demographic of organ donors, twenty-two people just like me, die every day waiting for one. This is not normal, and I will not accept it. I will rage against it. But I will rage myself to a ragged end if I don't assimilate these loses and these injustices into the story of my life. I'm just as much a heart patient as I am a transplant survivor, as I am former pastor and drummer, as I am an advocate for better health care, as I am a creative force for the betterment of our society.

Life goes on. The question is whether I will be able to go on with it, or whether I will stand in the dust and ashes of the catastrophe that visited me that day I ate the fish in 2010.

And if I don't go on with it, it is sure to drag me along one way or the other. I can even try to steer it in the direction I want it to go, but I know for certain that things outside of my control have a stronger hand on the wheel. No matter. This is what I've been given, and as much as I can choose what to do with it, I must.

There is no moral to the story. It's cliché', right? "Stuff happens." "It is what it is." "Maybe it's all for a reason." None of that helps.

At a particularly harrowing moment in their quest to save Middle Earth from the horrors of the One Ring, Frodo despairingly tells Gandalf the Wizard, "I wish the ring had never come to me… I wish none of this had ever happened."

"So do all who live to see such times," Gandalf tells him with a smile. "But all we can do is choose what to do with the time that is given to us."

And so we write songs that someone else might cling to in dark moments. And we write about our tragedies, our hopes, and the small victories we manage to tease out of it all so that someone else might find the strength to tie another knot in the rope, put one foot in front of the other, to eventually turn around. And we continue to get up each morning and figure out how to do the best we can with the time given to us. We fail, we disappoint the people around us, and more often, ourselves. But the alternative is to waste that time, the one thing that Helen Keller said, "can never be retrieved." She doesn't have to tell *me*.

Terry Pratchett once wrote, "The presence of those seeking the truth is infinitely to be preferred to the presence of those who think they've found it." (*Monstrous Regiment*) I spent my late teens, twenties, and early thirties being the latter, but now, having been "broken on the wheels of life" as Brennan Manning termed it, I'm convinced that I am the former. The trick for me is to not waste time trying so hard to find what that truth is that I forget to stop, look around, and live.

I could go on writing about this experience for the rest of my life, because it doesn't really ever end. It just starts to blend back into the time given to me. Not seamlessly, but with a jagged, roughly stitched edge that will carry over into the boy's lives and remain long after I'm gone. They're starting to realize that to a large degree, it has shaped who they are, and I see it every day in the way they handle crisis, disappointment, and pain, but also in how they plan, how they perceive others, and how they love. I lay the credit for that at their own feet, at Christie's feet, and at the feet of the people who collectively carried us through this when we could no longer walk or crawl.

It's taken me a year and half to write all of this, to craft the songs that would become its framework, and in a sense, it's added that time to the eighteen years from my original HCM diagnosis. I've written another letter to my donor's family on the second anniversary of the transplant, in hopes that they'll agree to hear Requiem for a Savior, at least. Maybe one day we'll meet. Maybe not. This has been simultaneously a cathartic and emotionally draining experience, and I'm more than ready to put most of it in a box on the closet shelf. I write this on the night before the book is submitted for publishing, knowing it will likely be the last time I'll have to re-read the account of that fateful day in Boston, that awful night in the ER in New Hampshire, the skin-of-our-teeth move to Pennsylvania, Perry's death, those thousands of laps on the HVI, or my long recovery. To continue dwelling on it is toxic, but to forget any would be a disservice to my donor, his family, my family, and to the others who didn't make it out alive. But I expect the farther away I am from it, the more I will smile instead of cry when I think about it all. In fact, I know I will.

I'm also certain that by now, I've talked and sang about it for quite long enough. So, I'm off to see what else I can do, and see, and become in the time my donor and my family have given me.

Conversations from Room 1170

Dave Johnson

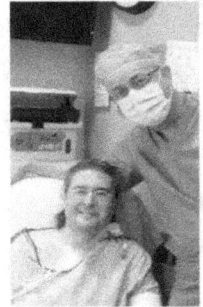
Dr. Behzad Soleimani

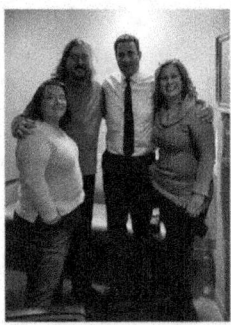
Christie, Dave,
Dr. Marty Maron, Lisa Salberg

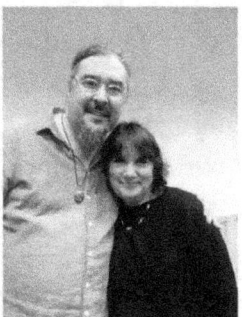
Fran Hrenko

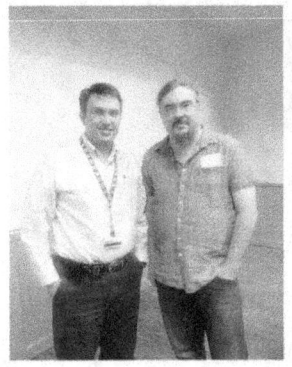
Dr. Eric Popjes

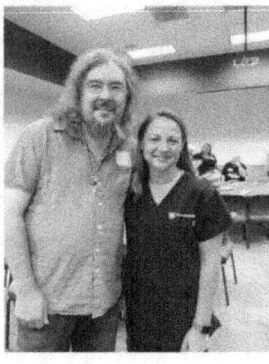
Tina Kline

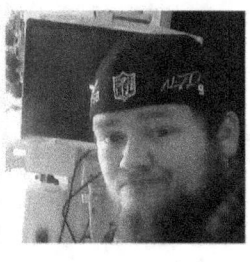
Perry Jenkins

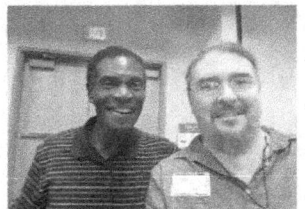
Dr. Dwight Davis

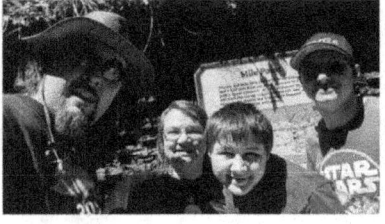
Dave, Christie, Brennan, Rich - Fall 2017

Conversations from Room 1170

Dave Johnson lives in Lebanon, Pennsylvania with his wife, two sons, and two dogs. He has written two full-length novels (under the pen name D.K. Johnson), The Ghost of Maddingbrew, a steampunk espionage tale for juvenile readers, and Lorenzo the Magnificent, an historical fiction story for young adult readers.

Conversations from Room 1170 is his first non-fiction, autobiographical work.

He's also a musician and songwriter. His fourth full-length double disc album is a companion to this book (also entitled Conversations from Room 1170) and features a song for each chapter of the story, written mostly during the time the events were taking place.

When not writing or recording, he homeschools his two boys, enjoys strategy board games (mostly Star Wars themed), volunteers with The Bodhana Group, a non-profit gaming therapy organization, and with Olivia's House (both based in York, PA) and serves as a patient advocate with the HCMA, Gift of Life, and the long-term care council at Penn State Hershey Med Center, where he received his donor heart.

For more information, find him on the web at www.davejohnsonstuff.com

www.ingramcontent.com/pod-product-compliance
Lightning Source LLC
Chambersburg PA
CBHW032210220526
45472CB00018B/664